Contents

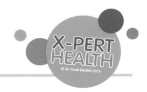

X-PERT Health is named after the clinical trial of the programme: E**X**pert **P**atient **E**ducation versus **R**outine **T**reatment. We are a registered charity who provide structured education programmes. The X-PERT Diabetes, X-PERT Insulin and X-PERT Prevention of Diabetes (X-POD) Programmes have been developed to help people self-manage their condition, and to improve their health and quality of life. All these programmes meet the key criteria identified by the Department of Health, Diabetes UK and the National Institute for Health and Care Excellence (NICE). The X-PERT Weight Programme is now also available, to help people lose fat and keep it off.

Although this handbook is not part of one of our programmes it has been developed based on the same principles. It uses the most recent scientific evidence to provide clear and useful information to those who might need it. A low carb dietary approach is very different to the lifestyle many people are used to. As a result they might need extra guidance and support to help them make meaningful changes. Finding a dietary approach that you can enjoy and are able to stick to is essential if you are going to achieve long-term success!

X-PERT programmes help people:

- reduce blood glucose levels, reduce blood pressure and improve the ratio of fats in their blood
- lose weight and reduce their waist size
- adopt a healthier dietary intake whilst also increasing enjoyment of food
- become more active
- reduce risk of developing future health problems
- increase confidence to look after health
- reduce depression and improve quality of life
- reduce prescribed medication

X-PERT Programmes are delivered throughout the UK & Ireland. For those who cannot attend a programme, or wish to re-cap on the information provided, a digital version is available. You can also visit the public shop on our website at www.xperthealth.org.uk.

If you would like to share your story or feedback, or if you have any questions, please email admin@xperthealth.org.uk

Sign up for the X-PERT newsletter and join our online forum, for free!

Email **admin@xperthealth.org.uk**, or go to our website, to sign up for the quarterly X-PERT newsletter; which will provide you with the latest information and useful tips.

You can also sign up to our online forum, at **www.xperthealth.org.uk/forums**, to receive ongoing support and ask any questions you might have about managing your health.

X-PERT Health is a charity (registration number: 1143561). Our mission is to enable all people at risk of, or diagnosed with, long-term conditions to receive good quality structured education that helps them to self-manage their condition leading to improved health and wellbeing. **If you would like to help us with our mission, either by helping us improve implementation in your area or by making a donation, please visit our website for more information.**

Connect with us through **f 𝕏 in** You**Tube** **◎** to hear about the latest news and research

What Is A Very Low Carb Lifestyle?

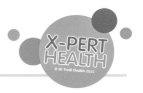

The dietary recommendations in the UK, and in much of the rest of the world, are based around a low fat lifestyle. Weight loss advice is often the same; to restrict calories by limiting the intake of fat. But for many people this approach is not successful. A low carb lifestyle is an alternative way of living, where you restrict the intake of carbs and instead get your energy by fuelling from healthy, natural fats.

But don't we need carbs?
The short answer is no! Our body only needs a very small amount of glucose, which is what carbs break down into. Our body is more than able to make enough glucose from fat or protein to fulfil these requirements. So the lower limit of how many carbs we NEED to consume is zero.

Aren't fats bad for me?
Fats have been demonised because they provide us with more energy gram-for-gram than carbs and proteins, and because they have been linked to cardiovascular disease. But this is unfair. Not all fats are the same, and if we get them from healthy, natural sources they are actually good for us. Although they are more energy dense than carbs, they are also very filling. So eating fats from the right sources means we are unlikely to overconsume them. You can read more about fats and how they affect our health on pages 70 to 73.

How low is "low" carb?
Although different definitions are sometimes used the most common definitions are:

- A **low carb** dietary approach contains fewer than 130g of carbs per day, or less than 26% total energy

- A **very low carb** dietary approach, the approach this handbook is based on, contains fewer than 50g carbs per day, or less than 10% energy

How do I know if it is right for me?
Many people who are overweight, or are normal weight but have a large waist size, have some level of insulin resistance (see pages 8 and 9). This means their body struggles to use glucose. If this is you, you may benefit from restricting your carb intake to some extent. There are also many people who experience other negative effects from eating too many carbs; for example digestive discomfort.

Some people just prefer the types of food that are encouraged as part of this dietary approach, 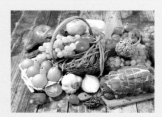 meaning they find it easier to follow and more enjoyable than a low fat diet. Anyone who has tried to follow a low fat lifestyle and has struggled to manage their weight and/or health may benefit from trying a different approach, and a very low carb lifestyle has been shown to be a safe and suitable alternative.

This handbook provides step-by-step instructions on how to follow a very low carb lifestyle; with practical advice, hints and tips to help you on the way.

Remember though, this is not a short-term solution, it is a lifestyle approach. The best dietary approach for an individual is whichever one they can stick to whilst still managing their health. This book sets out to help you find an approach that will work for **you** long-term.

This Dietary Approach Is Not A Quick Fix

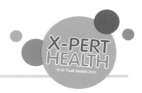

Almost any dietary approach can be effective in the short-term, but if people revert to their previous lifestyle it is likely that any benefits will be lost. Diets are frequently broken when the burden outweighs the benefit, and people start craving the foods they have been restricting. This usually leads to yo-yo dieting, with people re-gaining any weight they've lost and having worse health outcomes.

To prevent this happening it is important that any changes you make are sustainable, that they fit with your preferences, and that they lead to health improvements that can be maintained. You therefore need to adapt this dietary approach in a way that suits YOU.

People are more likely to sustain any dietary changes if they see some benefit, but changing the way you live your life is never easy. We are creatures of habit who generally like to keep things the way they are; so making changes can feel awkward or uncomfortable.

Old habits need to be replaced with new ones. This can take time, so you may need to be patient! A top tip is to make sure you enjoy what you eat. This will make your new lifestyle easier to stick to. If you can do this whilst eating a diverse range of REAL foods it is likely that you will be able to meet your body's nutritional requirements too. This will help further reduce cravings for other things, which will help you adopt this dietary approach long-term.

Questions to ask yourself before starting:

1. What do I hope to achieve from adopting a very low carb dietary approach?
....
....

2. How will I know if it is working for me?
....
....

3. What will I find easy?
....
....

4. What will I find difficult?
....
....

5. What could I do to obtain extra support?
....
....

6. How could I reduce or remove some of the barriers?
....
....

7. When would be a good time to start?
....
....

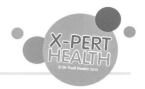

To help you understand why a very low carb dietary approach might work for you it is useful to understand what happens to different foods when you eat them.

The body needs 4 essential nutrients to keep healthy: fat, protein, vitamins and minerals. Water and fibre are not nutrients but they are also essential to life. Too much or too little of any of these essentials is not good for the body.

Carbohydrate (carb) is a nutrient, but it is NOT essential to life. This is because it doesn't provide us with anything we cannot get from other foods or that our body cannot make itself. Carbs are however important in relation to blood glucose control because it is the only nutrient that directly breaks down into glucose. All food and drink containing carbs releases glucose into the blood.

Glucose cannot be converted to energy until it enters a body cell. In response to raised blood glucose levels the pancreas (an organ in the body) produces a hormone called insulin. Insulin acts like a key, unlocking the door into the body cells. This allows the glucose to enter the cells to be used for energy.

However, many people are resistant to the effects of insulin. This means the insulin doesn't work as well, and the body has to produce more and more to try and compensate for this. This insulin resistance also means the body isn't able to deal with carbs as effectively. For more about insulin resistance see pages 8 and 9.

An introduction to carbs:

There are **2 types of carb foods...**

1. Starchy foods

For example:
Potatoes, Rice, Pasta, Bread, Breakfast Cereal, Porridge, Chapattis, Crackers

2. Food containing sugar

Added sugar:
Sugar, Jam, Honey, Fizzy Drinks, Sweets, Cakes, Biscuits, Desserts

Natural sugar:
Fruit, Milk, Yoghurt

BREAD

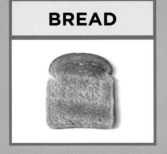

SUGAR

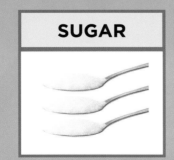

APPLE

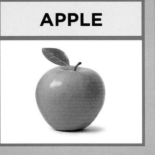

MILK

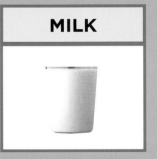

Our body breaks these foods down into **Glucose (◯),** which goes into our...

...BLOOD...

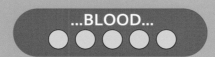

...and can be taken to the body cells to be used for **ENERGY**

What Happens To Food When We Eat It?

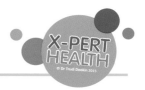

We get most of our energy from carbs, fat or protein. These are called macronutrients. How our body digests these macronutrients is described on this page and the next.

As mentioned previously carbs are not essential to life, and they are the only nutrient that directly increases blood glucose levels. Restricting carbs can therefore help to reduce blood glucose and, as a result, insulin levels. As elevated insulin can lead to insulin resistance and problems

managing weight and health, restricting carbs can help address these issues.

If you omit carbs from your diet you will start to use dietary and stored body fat as fuel instead of glucose. Your body will become more efficient at burning fat rather than storing it, helping with energy levels and weight management. There are a number of other possible benefits from following a very low carb dietary approach, which are discussed on pages 10 to 12.

Carb digestion

1. Carbs are broken down into glucose, fructose, and galactose in the gut

2. Glucose is absorbed from the gut and increases blood glucose levels. The normal range of blood glucose is 3.5 to 7.8 mmol/l

3. Fructose and galactose go to the liver where they are either stored* or converted to glucose to be used for energy

4. Insulin is released and acts as a key to unlock the cell door so that the glucose can enter the cell

5. Once in the cell the glucose can be converted to energy

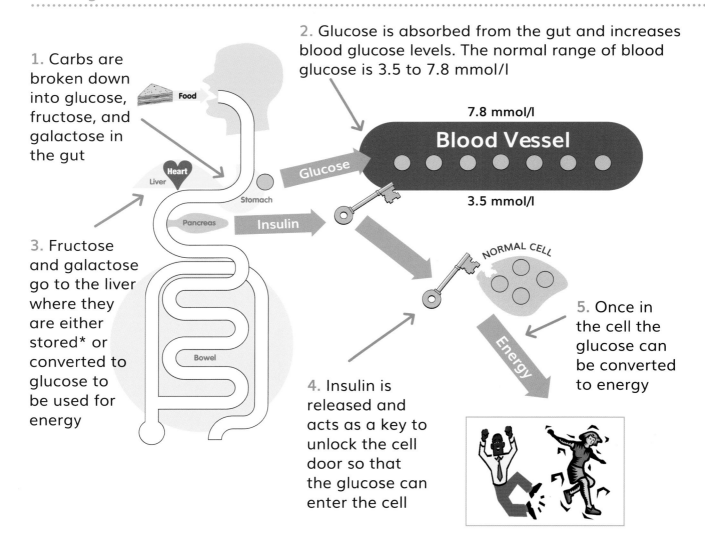

* they can either be stored as glycogen, a carb reserve, or be converted to and stored as fat. The body only has limited space to store glycogen

What Happens To Food When We Eat It?

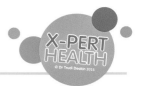

Protein digestion

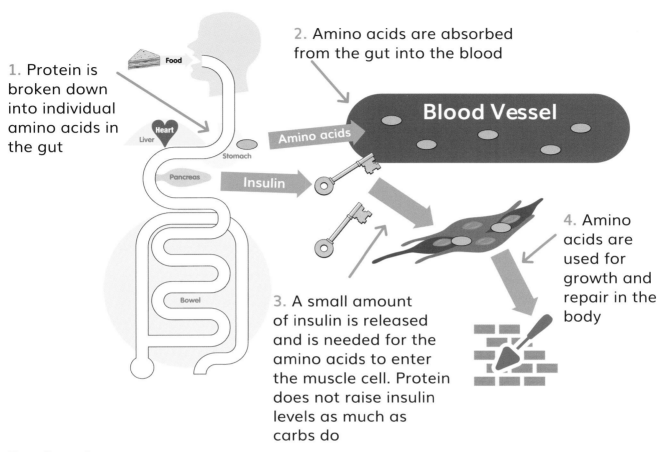

1. Protein is broken down into individual amino acids in the gut

2. Amino acids are absorbed from the gut into the blood

Blood Vessel

Amino acids

Insulin

4. Amino acids are used for growth and repair in the body

3. A small amount of insulin is released and is needed for the amino acids to enter the muscle cell. Protein does not raise insulin levels as much as carbs do

Fat digestion

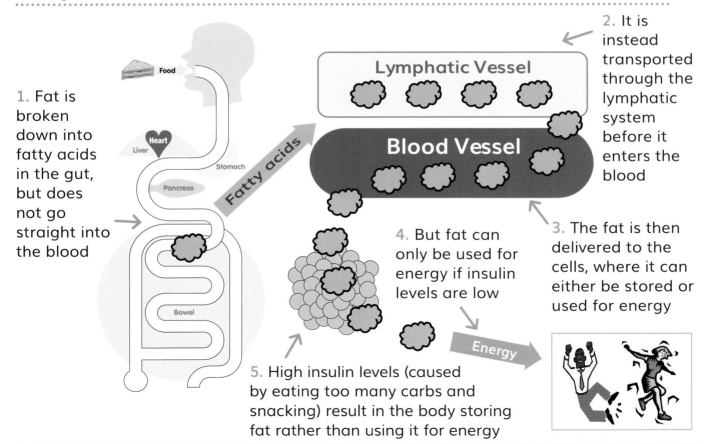

1. Fat is broken down into fatty acids in the gut, but does not go straight into the blood

Lymphatic Vessel

Fatty acids

Blood Vessel

2. It is instead transported through the lymphatic system before it enters the blood

3. The fat is then delivered to the cells, where it can either be stored or used for energy

4. But fat can only be used for energy if insulin levels are low

Energy

5. High insulin levels (caused by eating too many carbs and snacking) result in the body storing fat rather than using it for energy

Insulin Resistance

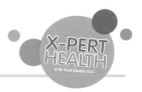

What is insulin resistance?

We need insulin to allow glucose to enter our body cells. Insulin resistance is a condition whereby the body cells fail to respond to the normal actions of insulin, i.e. the insulin key struggles to unlock the door into the cell. As a result, for any given amount of glucose more insulin is needed to help it into the cells.

Why is insulin resistance a problem?

When our insulin doesn't work properly it becomes more difficult for our body to keep blood glucose levels in a healthy range. More insulin is released to compensate for this, which leads to our body storing fat rather than burning it. This makes it more difficult to manage our weight, which can contribute to a number health issues.

What causes insulin resistance?

There are a number of possible causes, including:

1. Excess fat stored in our cells can make them resistant to the effects of insulin

2. Increased frequency of eating, and consumption of a large amount of quick-releasing carbs in particular, can cause repeated surges in blood glucose. This results in continuous high levels of insulin (hyperinsulinaemia), which can cause insulin resistance. This is similar to how antibiotic resistance occurs: a high exposure to antibiotics can lead to bacteria becoming resistant to their effects

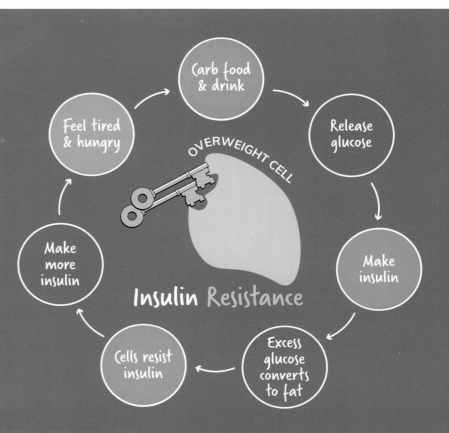

Vicious cycles

Both of the main causes of insulin resistance mentioned above, excess fat storage and overexposure to insulin, can lead to cycles that cause further insulin resistance if we don't do anything to address them. This is because when we are insulin resistant the insulin we do have doesn't work as well, which means we need to produce more insulin to do the same job. This rise in insulin will lead to a further increase in fat storage and greater exposure to insulin, which - as explained above - both increase insulin resistance!

Another vicious cycle is outlined in the figure above. When we consume carbs blood glucose and insulin levels rise. Any excess glucose is stored as fat and, because insulin levels are increased, any fat in our diet is stored too. Over time this increases insulin resistance, causing even higher insulin levels. High insulin levels keep us in fat storage mode, and insulin resistance means we can't use glucose efficiently. The body therefore can't access enough energy, and we feel tired and hungry as a result. This leads us to crave more carbs, which starts this cycle again.

Insulin Resistance

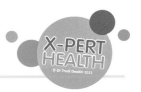

Can I reduce insulin resistance?

Insulin resistance is an important issue that, if unaddressed, can lead to long-term health problems. It is possible to reduce insulin resistance though, for example by:

1. **reducing carb intake.** This is the primary focus of this handbook as carbs are the main driver of elevated insulin levels

2. **swapping quick releasing carbs for slower releasing carbs** (see page 101). Slower releasing carbs can reduce surges in blood glucose and insulin levels

3. **intermittent fasting** (see pages 48 to 51). When we have spells without eating our insulin levels drop. Omitting snacks can be a simple way to ensure there are periods of the day where your insulin levels are not raised

4. **losing weight.** Any method of losing body fat (especially from the waist) will help to reduce insulin resistance, though it is important that this can be sustained long-term

5. **increasing physical activity levels,** as muscle contractions help glucose enter the cells without the need for as much insulin

How do I know if I have insulin resistance?

Most people who struggle to manage their weight have some level of insulin resistance. There are blood tests that can assess how much insulin you are making, and the degree of insulin resistance can be calculated from blood glucose and insulin test results. Insulin measurement is not currently included in the standard tests undertaken by your GP however. Assessing whether someone has the metabolic syndrome (see box to the right) is a good proxy measure of this though, as it is strongly associated with insulin resistance.

Metabolic syndrome

The metabolic syndrome is defined as having three or more of the risk factors below. For more information about these risk factors, and other indicators of health, see pages 109 to 112. The international cut points are:

Increased waist size: Greater than 94cm in Caucasian men and greater than 80cm in Caucasian women, or greater than 90cm in South Asian men and greater than 80cm South Asian women

Raised triglycerides: Greater than 1·7mmol/l (or on medication to reduce triglycerides)

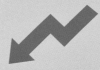

Reduced HDL-cholesterol: Less than 1·0mmol/l in men; less than 1·3mmol/l in women

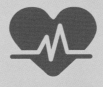

Raised blood pressure: Systolic greater than 130 mmHg; Diastolic greater than 85mmHg (or on medication to reduce blood pressure)

Raised fasting glucose: Fasting plasma glucose greater than 5·6mmol/l

Possible Benefits Of Reducing Carb Intake

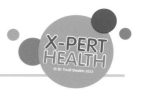

As well as an ability to reduce insulin and insulin resistance, there is emerging evidence that a very low carb lifestyle may have a number of other benefits. It may even help to treat or reduce the risk of a number of other health conditions. These include:

A reduction in appetite

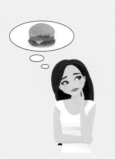

One common reason for a diet failing is hunger. A benefit of the reduced carb approach is that it can lead to a reduction in appetite and less frequent eating. This may be because we are better able to access our body's stored fat when our insulin levels are reduced, or because the real foods encouraged on this dietary approach are more filling and meet our nutritional requirements better than the types of food many people usually eat.

Fat loss and weight reduction

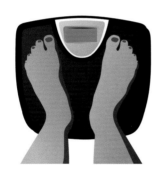

Reducing carb intake can be an effective way to lose body weight. The body can adapt and become efficient at burning body fat instead of storing it. Fat can become the preferred fuel for energy, which is good news as most people have a surplus of it! Using body fat for fuel can also lead to increased energy levels, without the dips that high carb intakes can cause (e.g. daytime sleepiness or tiredness). A very low carb dietary approach can be effective at reducing abdominal (belly) fat, which can decrease insulin resistance and risk of cardiovascular disease (CVD).

Reduced blood pressure

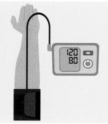

High blood pressure is one of the main modifiable risk factors for CVD. Lowering blood pressure is therefore considered a very important step to reduce this risk. Multiple studies have demonstrated that restricting carbs can lead to a reduction in blood pressure.

Improved blood lipid profile

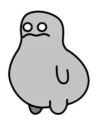

When carbs are reduced this often leads to a reduction in blood fat (triglyceride) levels and the number of small, unstable low density lipoprotein (LDL) particles; whilst increasing consumption of healthy fats can raise levels of HDL cholesterol (see pages 110 and 111 for more information about these health indicators). These factors have all been linked to a reduced risk of CVD.

Improve skin problems and slow signs of aging

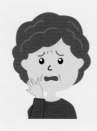

Many skin problems and signs of aging are related to inflammation and oxidative stress, which can be reduced on a very low carb dietary approach. Elevated insulin can also cause an increase in oil production in the skin, which can lead to pimples forming. Therefore reducing insulin by restricting carbs can help.

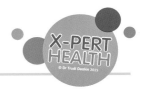

A reduction in prescribed medication

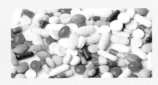

If you are on prescribed medication you may be able to significantly reduce (or even omit) this, as reducing carbs can potentially help improve some of the symptoms you are taking medication for. This is particularly evident in people with diabetes, where restricting carbs can dramatically reduce the need for blood glucose controlling medications such as insulin. It is very important to discuss any medication changes with your healthcare team so that it can be adjusted appropriately.

A reduction in CVD risk

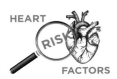

The National Institute for Health and Care Excellence (NICE) guidance states that people over 40 years of age should have their cardiovascular disease (CVD) risk reviewed frequently. Some risk factors such as age, sex, and family history cannot be modified, but others such as weight and blood pressure can. Having elevated insulin levels is also associated with an increased risk of CVD. Reducing carbs can help improve many of these factors, as discussed previously, and thus can reduce the risk of CVD.

Improvement in liver function

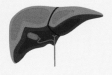

The liver has many important functions in the body. A healthy liver should contain little or no fat, yet 25-30% of people have an early form of non-alcoholic fatty liver disease (NAFLD). One of the main causes of fatty liver is the overconsumption of carbs, particularly sugary carbs. This is because they are processed by the liver and any excess is converted to and stored as fat. Reducing carb intake can therefore help reduce the amount of fat in the liver.

Reduced inflammation

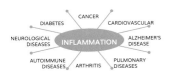

Inflammation is an important process to help the body deal with short-term damage, but many people have a lifestyle that leads to long-term inflammation. This chronic inflammation is an important factor in the development of many conditions, including CVD. Insulin resistance and blood glucose spikes have been shown to increase long-term inflammation. There is evidence that reducing carb intake can lower levels of C-Reactive Protein (CRP), indicating reduced inflammation.

Reduced irritable bowel syndrome (IBS) symptoms

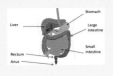

IBS is one of the most common gut disorders, affecting up to 20% of the population. Common symptoms include bloating, abdominal pain, and bouts of diarrhoea and/or constipation. Reducing carbs may help reduce pain, improve stool habits and improve quality of life in IBS sufferers.

Possible Benefits Of Reducing Carb Intake

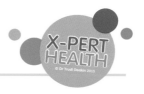

Improvements in heartburn and acid reflux

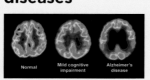

Heartburn and acid reflux symptoms are common complaints affecting up to 40% of adults. Heartburn is defined as a burning sensation, whereas acid reflux is when some of the contents of the stomach is pushed back into the food pipe. Reducing carb intake can help to resolve these symptoms in some people.

A possible treatment, or prevention, for neurological and neurodegenerative diseases

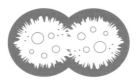

This dietary approach has been used as an effective epileptic seizure treatment, especially in children. Recent reports have suggested that adopting a very low carb dietary approach may provide relief for, slow progression of, or potentially lead to improvements related to several neurological conditions including Alzheimer's, Parkinson's, multiple sclerosis, mental health disorders (e.g. bipolar disorder) and traumatic brain injury. Research is still in its infancy but people may benefit from dedicated intensive and tailored treatment to reduce insulin resistance and obtain target blood glucose and blood pressure control.

A possible treatment for cancer

It has been suggested that a reduced carb intake, alongside other therapies, could help slow the progression of some cancers. Normal cells can use glucose, fat or ketones for fuel; but many cancer cells thrive exclusively on glucose. Cancer cell growth may therefore be suppressed by 1) consuming very few carbs, as this may reduce energy availability, and 2) lowering insulin levels. Work on this is in the early stages however, and much more research is needed.

Possible benefits specific to women

Improvements in polycystic ovary syndrome (PCOS) symptoms

PCOS is a common condition, affecting millions of women, that is associated with insulin resistance. Tiny cysts develop in the ovaries, affecting the way they work. Symptoms of PCOS include irregular periods, increased body hair, weight gain, acne and fertility problems. Reducing insulin levels, by reducing carb consumption, can help to improve symptoms and may even be able to remove the condition altogether.

A reduction in premenstrual tension (PMT) symptoms

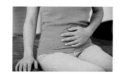

PMT is believed to affect approximately 80% of women and is used to describe a wide range of symptoms which occur after the middle of the menstrual cycle (ovulation) and disappear almost as soon as the period arrives. Symptoms can range from bloating, breast tenderness, migraines, depression, mood swings and food cravings. Symptoms may be eased by reducing carb intake.

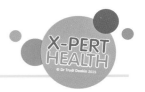

Nutritional Ketosis

When following a very low carb dietary approach some people will enter a state called nutritional ketosis. There is often confusion around ketones, with many people associating them with a very serious condition that can occur in people with type 1 diabetes (predominantly). These concerns are misplaced however.

What are ketones?

Ketones are produced when fat is burned for energy. They are a natural product which can provide an excellent source of energy, especially for the brain. Ketones are more likely to be produced when carb consumption is restricted or when fasting, because under these conditions the body turns to using fat as its primary source of energy.

Are ketones dangerous?

No. Although some people worry about being in nutritional ketosis because they have heard that ketones are bad for you this is simply not true. The only time ketones are harmful is when they are produced in abundance when people with type 1 diabetes have insufficient insulin and high blood glucose levels - a condition called diabetic ketoacidosis (DKA).

What is the difference between nutritional ketosis and DKA?

In nutritional ketosis both blood glucose and insulin levels are low, whilst blood ketones are slightly raised. This reflects that fat is being used as the main source of energy. Growing children, pregnant women and anyone on a weight reducing diet can make ketones; though for most people carb intake needs to be consistently lower than 50g per day to remain in nutritional ketosis.

DKA however is a serious condition where ketone levels AND blood glucose levels are dramatically raised. It is these extreme levels of both ketones and glucose, in the presence of insulin insufficiency and dehydration, that results in DKA.

Is nutritional ketosis a good thing?

Research has shown a number of benefits from being in nutritional ketosis, many of which are related to the restriction of carbs and subsequent lowering of insulin levels. See pages 10 to 12 for a summary of some of these benefits.

So what should my ketone levels be?

If you are in nutritional ketosis your ketone levels should be between 0.5 and 3.0 mmol/l, though some people report having values that are slightly higher than this (closer to 5.0 mmol/l).

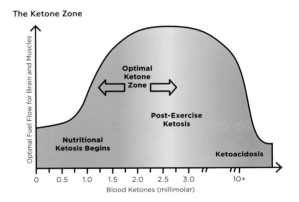

How can I measure my ketone levels?

If you are achieving your health goals, it is not necessary to measure ketone levels. However, if you would like to, there are three ways to test:

- urine test strips
- home blood meters
- breath test meters

Urine test strips measure the level of a ketone called acetoacetate in the urine. However, once your body has adapted to burning fat for energy urine testing may not be as accurate. Many blood meters will measure levels of beta-hydroxybutyrate (BHB) and although the meters are not expensive the test strips can be. The breath test measures acetone in the breath that is released after burning BHB for energy.

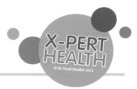

This section of the handbook will go through six practical steps to help you adopt, and adapt to, a very low carb dietary approach. These steps are designed to help you change your current dietary approach into one that you can enjoy whilst also improving your health.

Before starting you need to determine the sources and amount of carbs in your current diet. This will help you work out what changes you need to make.

The next 7 pages have blank food diaries to allow you to record everything you eat for an entire week. Simply write down everything you have at each meal, or as snacks, including how much of it you have (this can either be a rough estimate, or you can measure things more accurately if you prefer).

Tip: sometimes it can be difficult to remember everything you have eaten during the day, so it may help if you keep a record of what you are eating as you go through the day.

Example of (part of) a completed food diary:

Lunch:
Baked potato (200g, cooked)
Salad: lettuce (handful), tomato (x1), cucumber (3cm chunk)
Grated cheese (30g)
Baked beans (1 small tin)
Evening Meal:
Chicken fillet (150g uncooked)
Pasta spiral, white (250g cooked)
Tomato, chopped (1 tin)
Mixed vegetables: Sweetcorn (1 tablespoon), Broccoli (1 tablespoon)
Snacks: morning, afternoon and evening (if consumed in addition to meals)
Banana (1, medium sized)
Coffee with semi-skimmed milk and 1 teaspoon sugar

Step 1: What Are You Currently Eating?

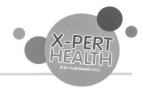

Date ....

Write down everything you eat and drink during day 1. The information from this food diary will be used in the next step.

Breakfast:

Lunch:

Evening Meal:

Snacks: morning, afternoon and evening (if consumed in addition to meals)

Supper:

N.B. If you found it helpful to keep a food diary you might like to record your food intake more frequently either by writing it in a notebook or using an internet or phone app such as My Fitness Pal™. Blank food diary templates can also be downloaded from our free online forum, accessible at **www.xperthealth.org.uk/forums**.

Step 1: What Are You Currently Eating?

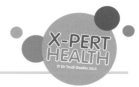

Date ....

Write down everything you eat and drink during day 2.
The information from this food diary will be used in the next step.

Breakfast:

_____

_____

_____

_____

Lunch:

_____

_____

_____

_____

Evening Meal:

_____

_____

_____

_____

Snacks: morning, afternoon and evening (if consumed in addition to meals)

_____

_____

_____

_____

Supper:

_____

_____

_____

N.B. If you found it helpful to keep a food diary you might like to record your food intake more frequently either by writing it in a notebook or using an internet or phone app such as My Fitness Pal™. Blank food diary templates can also be downloaded from our free online forum, accessible at www.xperthealth.org.uk/forums.

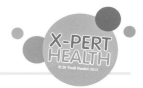

Date ....

> Write down everything you eat and drink during day 3.
> The information from this food diary will be used in the next step.

Breakfast:

Lunch:

Evening Meal:

Snacks: morning, afternoon and evening (if consumed in addition to meals)

Supper:

N.B. If you found it helpful to keep a food diary you might like to record your food intake more frequently either by writing it in a notebook or using an internet or phone app such as My Fitness Pal™. Blank food diary templates can also be downloaded from our free online forum, accessible at **www.xperthealth.org.uk/forums**.

Step 1: What Are You Currently Eating?

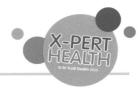

Date ....

Write down everything you eat and drink during day 4.
The information from this food diary will be used in the next step.

Breakfast:

Lunch:

Evening Meal:

Snacks: morning, afternoon and evening (if consumed in addition to meals)

Supper:

N.B. If you found it helpful to keep a food diary you might like to record your food intake more frequently either by writing it in a notebook or using an internet or phone app such as My Fitness Pal™. Blank food diary templates can also be downloaded from our free online forum, accessible at **www.xperthealth.org.uk/forums**.

Step 1: What Are You Currently Eating?

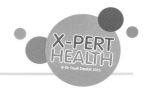

Date ....

Write down everything you eat and drink during day 5. The information from this food diary will be used in the next step.

Breakfast:

Lunch:

Evening Meal:

Snacks: morning, afternoon and evening (if consumed in addition to meals)

Supper:

N.B. If you found it helpful to keep a food diary you might like to record your food intake more frequently either by writing it in a notebook or using an internet or phone app such as My Fitness Pal™. Blank food diary templates can also be downloaded from our free online forum, accessible at **www.xperthealth.org.uk/forums**.

Step 1: What Are You Currently Eating?

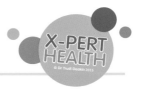

Date ....

> Write down everything you eat and drink during day 6.
> The information from this food diary will be used in the next step.

Breakfast:

Lunch:

Evening Meal:

Snacks: morning, afternoon and evening (if consumed in addition to meals)

Supper:

N.B. If you found it helpful to keep a food diary you might like to record your food intake more frequently either by writing it in a notebook or using an internet or phone app such as My Fitness Pal™. Blank food diary templates can also be downloaded from our free online forum, accessible at www.xperthealth.org.uk/forums.

Step 1: What Are You Currently Eating?

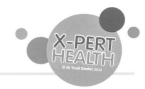

Date ....

> Write down everything you eat and drink during day 7.
> The information from this food diary will be used in the next step.

Breakfast:

Lunch:

Evening Meal:

Snacks: morning, afternoon and evening (if consumed in addition to meals)

Supper:

N.B. If you found it helpful to keep a food diary you might like to record your food intake more frequently either by writing it in a notebook or using an internet or phone app such as My Fitness Pal™. Blank food diary templates can also be downloaded from our free online forum, accessible at **www.xperthealth.org.uk/forums**.

Step 2: Identifying Carb Containing Foods

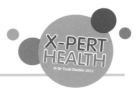

Once you have recorded what you eat during a normal week (see step 1) you can then identify what sources of carbs you have in your diet. Doing this makes it easier to work out what needs removing or replacing, and helps you consider what you might want to replace it with. Highlight or circle the foods and drinks that contain carbs in the food diaries you completed during step 1.

The following sections of this handbook can help you identify which foods and drinks contain carbs:

- Examples of Carb-Containing Foods (page 23)
- Foods that contain little, moderate or high carbs (pages 24 to 26)
- Alcohol (page 79)
- Carb Content of Everyday Foods (pages 91 to 100)

Example of (part of) a completed food diary, with carb containing foods circled:

Lunch:

Baked potato (200g, cooked)

Salad: lettuce (handful), tomato (x1), cucumber (3cm chunk)

Grated cheese (30g)

Baked beans (1 small tin)

Evening Meal:

Chicken fillet (150g uncooked)

Pasta spirals, white (250g cooked)

Tomato, chopped (1 tin)

Mixed vegetables: Sweetcorn (1 tablespoon), Broccoli (1 tablespoon)

Snacks: morning, afternoon and evening (if consumed in addition to meals)

Banana (1, medium sized)

Coffee with semi-skimmed milk and 1 sugar

Please note: salad ingredients and mixed vegetables have not been circled, even though they contain small amounts of carbs. However, if eaten to excess or in a concentrated form (e.g. chopped tomatoes) they can still add a significant amount of carbs

Step 2: Identifying Carb Containing Foods

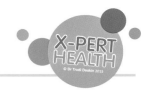

Many popular foods are high in carbs. The table below includes examples of carb-based foods and drinks. These will need to be reduced or removed from your diet if you wish to reduce your carb consumption to less than 50g per day.

Breakfast

 Cereal & Milk

 Bread

 Crumpets

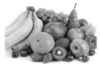 Fruit

 Yoghurt

 Jam/ Marmalade

Lunch and evening meal

 Bread, Chapatti & Naan

 Potato

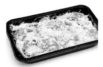 Takeaway & Ready Meals

 Pie

 Chips

 Pasta & Sauce

 Rice

 Pulses

 Battered Chicken or Fish

Plus very small amounts of carbs in salad and vegetables

Drinks

 Juice

 Milk

 Sugar in Drinks

 Fizzy Drinks

 Malted Drinks

 Alcoholic Drinks

Snacks and desserts

 Biscuits & Scones

 Fresh & Dried Fruit

 Yoghurt & Ice Cream

 Cakes & Muffins

 Sweets

 Puddings & Custards

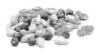 Nuts

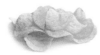 Crisps

 Chocolate

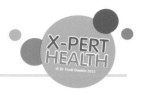

Once you have identified all of the carb containing foods you are currently eating (step 2) you need to consider which of these need omitting. A very low carb dietary approach contains less than 50g of carbs per day, so it is important to omit any foods that have a high carb content. If you omit all starch and sugar rich food and drink then it is more likely that you will meet this target.

The following tables include foods high in carbs that need to be eliminated on a very low carb diet ("red light" foods). These foods contain more than 10g carbs *per portion*.

Starches:

All breakfast cereals, bread (including gluten free), baps, finger roll, baguette, bagel, muffin, crumpet, fruit tea cake, potato (boiled, baked, mash, chips, French fries), rice, pasta, ravioli, noodles (egg & rice), vermicelli, gnocchi, chapatti, naan, paratha, roti, brioche, croissant, pain au chocolat, couscous, crackers & crispbread, croutons, ciabatta, panini, focaccia, pitta bread, flatbread, tortilla, poppadom, pancakes, waffle, hot cross bun, scones, rice cakes, dumplings, Yorkshire pudding, stuffing, hash brown, potato croquette, yam, bulgur wheat, quinoa, polenta

Vegetables:

Sweet potato, parsnips, plantain, sweetcorn, beetroot

Fruit:

Apple, orange, banana, grapes, plums, dried fruit (dates, figs, prunes, raisins, sultanas), tinned fruit, grapes, mango, melon, persimmon, peach, pear, pineapple, banana chips

Dairy:

Yoghurt with added sugar and fruit, custard, milk pudding, milkshake, oat milk

Protein:

Note: meat, fish and eggs do not contain carbs, but legumes and nuts do. Many processed protein foods combine protein with carbs though

Pulses - mushy peas, baked beans, butter & kidney beans, chickpeas, lentils. Meat, poultry or fish coated in batter or breadcrumbs (e.g. chicken kiev, fish fingers, battered fish, calamari), scotch egg, savoury pies & sausage rolls, haggis, seafood sticks, cashew & soya nuts

Fats, sweets & condiments/sauces:

Note: most natural fatty foods do not contain carbs, but baked and processed foods often combine fats with carbs

All desserts & puddings, sweet pies, biscuits, cakes, sweets, chocolate, confectionery, ice cream, sorbet, jelly, mousse, crisps, bombay mix, popcorn, pretzels, tortilla chips, prawn crackers, jam, marmalade, honey, syrup, lemon curd, chocolate spread, sugar, chutney, tomato, brown & chilli sauce

Ready meals or takeaways:

Pizza, burgers, bhaji, spring roll, samosa, pakora, any meals that include: pasta, potato, rice, bread (e.g. chapatti, naan)

Beverages:

Sugar and/or syrup added to coffee/ tea, cappuccino, latte, hot chocolate, all fruit juices, smoothie, sugar-sweetened cordial & fizzy drinks. Alcohol (see pages 78 and 79) - sweet wines & liqueurs, cider, alcopops, ale & carb-rich lager & beer

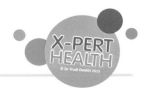

As well as the "red light" foods to avoid listed on the previous page there are a number of foods that should only be eaten in moderation ("amber light" foods). These foods contain small amounts of carbs (2g to 10g *per portion*) but, if eaten to excess, could result in your total carb intake exceeding the 50g target.

Starches:

Flour substitutes such as ground almonds, coconut flour, and soya flour

Vegetables:

Peas, bean sprouts, brussel sprouts, butternut squash, carrots, mangetout, onion, coleslaw, soup (fresh, tinned or homemade without starch filler), gherkins, pickled onion

Fruit:

Berries (strawberries, raspberries, blueberries, blackberries, black/redcurrants), cherries, apricot, nectarine, clementine, satsuma, fig, kiwi, papaya or plum, pomegranate, grapefruit, rhubarb (no added sugar), tomato (fresh, tinned, sun-dried)

Dairy:

Full fat milk, full fat natural yoghurt, coconut milk, unsweetened soya milk, raita

Protein:

Black pudding, sausages, pâté, BBQ ribs (depending on what sauce is used). Whole nuts (almonds, Brazil, hazelnuts, macadamia, peanuts, pecan, pistachio, walnuts, pine nuts), ground almonds, seeds, Marmite™, peanut butter, houmous, Quorn™

Fats, sweets & condiments/sauces:

Desserts, puddings, cakes & biscuits made with flour substitutes, low carb sweeteners and chocolate with greater than 70% cocoa. Gravy made with granules. Sauce (horseradish, mint, roux, piccalilli, soy, tartare, Worcestershire), salad cream and full fat salad dressing. Cream (single, whipping, clotted or soured) and crème fraÎche

Ready meals or takeaways:

Meat, fish and vegetable based dishes without rice, pasta, potato or bread. The following may be sufficiently low carb: Indian curries without rice, chapatti or naan; Chinese stir-fry without rice or noodles; kebabs with salad and without the pitta bread, and sushi containing a small amount of rice

Beverages:

Milk in coffee/tea, dry white wine, red wine, champagne, some brands of beer/lager (see alcohol section on pages 78 and 79 for more information)

The carb content of many common foods is included on pages 91 to 100. These pages also include information about how much of these foods would be considered to be a portion, so they can help you identify which foods you may want to include or omit as part of your new dietary approach.

There are other resources available to help you assess the carb content of different foods/drinks. The Carbs & Cals book and mobile phone app are popular options, providing a visual guide of the carb content of different serving sizes of a large number of foods. You can find out more at **www.carbsandcals.com**

Step 4: What Can You Eat?

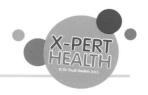

In step 3 you considered what foods should be limited or omitted when following a low carb dietary approach. Step 4 is to look at foods which can be consumed more freely.

It is essential that you identify foods you enjoy to include regularly. If you enjoy your dietary approach you are much more likely to stick to it. The table below includes foods that contain virtually no carbs ("green light" foods). These foods should make up to bulk of your new dietary approach.

Starches:

Starches are rich in carbs so need omitting (see red light box on page 24). Any flour substitute such as ground almonds, golden milled flaxseed, psyllium husk, coconut flour or soya flour can be eaten in moderation (see amber light box on page 25)

Vegetables:

Asparagus, aubergine, bamboo shoots, broad beans, broccoli, cabbage, cauliflower, celeriac, celery, courgette, cucumber, garlic, green beans, leeks, lettuce, mushrooms, okra, pak choi, peppers, rocket, spinach, spring greens, swede, turnip, watercress

Fruit:

All fruit contains carbs and so needs to be portion controlled (see amber light box on page 25) or avoided (see red light box on page 24). Avocado and olives can however be consumed more freely

Dairy:

Cheese - all types and varieties except those with added fruit such as apricots and cranberries, almond milk

Protein:

All meat, poultry, fish & seafood; including meats that have undergone some (but not excessive) processing, such as high meat content (~98%) sausages & beef burgers, chorizo, pancetta, parma ham, prosciutto, salami and pork scratchings. Eggs (boiled, scrambled, fried, poached, omelette), tofu

Fats, sweets & condiments/sauces:

Olive, coconut & palm oil, cold-pressed rapeseed oil, butter, lard, mayonnaise (full fat), double cream, low carb sweeteners (see pages 76 and 77), gravy made with meat juices, sauces (bearnaise, hollandaise, cream), mustard, pesto

Ready meal or takeaways:

Meat or fish sashimi, and many supermarkets or food outlets now provide pre-packed low carb options

Beverages:

Black coffee or tea, artificially sweetened cordial and sugar-free fizzy drinks

Alcohol - spirits such as vodka, gin, rum & whiskey do not contain carbs but need to be mixed with sugar-free drinks and consumed within government recommendations (see pages 78 and 79)

When reducing carb intake it is important to eat sufficient fat to satisfy your appetite. **But remember, reducing carb intake will make it easier for your body to use its own fat stores for energy, which can account for some of the "high fat" part of this dietary approach!** To meet your dietary requirements it is recommended to consume 5 to 10 portions of dietary fat each day (see page 27). Further information about dietary fat can be found on pages 70 to 73.

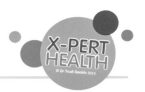

Step 4: What Can You Eat?

The Nutrition for Health Model below gives an outline of how many portions* from each food group are recommended for someone following a very low carb dietary approach. It also discusses why we do (or don't) need to include foods from each of these groups. The ranges presented are just a guide, and different people will have different individual requirements. Green light foods, those included in the table on page 26, should make up most of these portions, and there are some useful hints and tips on pages 42 to 47.

Following the Nutrition for Health guidance will provide all the essential nutrients: fat, protein, vitamins and minerals, and fibre**. Water is also an essential component: so aim to drink 1 to 2 litres per day, to thirst.

Most food and drink provide some of the essentials for life, but to obtain the best nutrition it is better to prepare and eat fresh unprocessed food rather than rely on convenience food or ready meals.

Fruit & vegetables
5-9 Portions

Provide a variety of vitamins and minerals, fibre and antioxidants and can help prevent illness and reduce the risk of future health problems

Carbs
0 Portions

Although carbs can provide energy and fibre we can get these from other food sources.

🍔 Processed Foods

Most highly processed foods are not good for you (see pages 74 and 75), so avoid them

Proteins
2-4 Portions

Essential for growth and repair of the body. They also provide essential vitamins and minerals, e.g. red meat is a good source of iron

Dairy
2-3 Portions

Provide vitamins and minerals, including calcium which is essential for healthy bones and teeth

Fats
5-10 Portions

Essential to life, and most of your energy will come from fat on this dietary approach. There are natural, healthy fats that are good for us and processed fats that can cause ill health (see pages 70 to 73)

* Information about what constitutes a portion can be found on page 31
** For more information about dietary fibre see pages 102 and 103

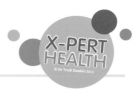

Step 4: What Can You Eat?

To provide you with ideas of what to eat, and how the information on pages 26 and 27 might translate into actual meals, there are 7-days of suggestions for meals and snacks over the next two pages. Mix and match these options to find an approach that suits you.

Most people find that their appetite reduces when adopting a very low carb dietary approach, and so they only need to eat on one to three occasions each day. Remember that it can take some time to adjust to change though, so if you usually eat three meals plus snacks it might take a little time to fully adjust to a new eating pattern.

7-day breakfast ideas

Day 1		Bacon, eggs, sausages*, fried mushroom, ½ fried tomato and butter (for frying)
Day 2		Scrambled eggs made with butter & a variety of additions such as cheese, onion or fish
Day 3		Fried kippers or mackerel with tomato
Day 4		Avocado with smoked salmon
Day 5		Berries with full fat Greek yoghurt or cream
Day 6		Omelette with a variety of fillings
Day 7		Bacon sandwich with low carb bread (see recipe for English muffin on page 86)

*make sure they have a high meat content, as some sausages with lower meat content actually include a lot of carbs. Generally speaking, higher meat content also means the product is less highly processed

Snacks and desserts (although we generally recommend omitting snacks, the examples below are better choices if you decide you do want a snack or wish to replace a meal)

Day 1	Hard cheese	Olives
Day 2	Full fat natural Greek yoghurt	Low carb chocolate cake (see recipes on pages 85 and 90)
Day 3	Dark bitter chocolate (70 - 100% cocoa solids)	Nuts
Day 4	Ground almond & walnut scones (see recipe on page 86)	Cucumber with full fat sour cream or tzatziki
Day 5	Pork scratchings	Cold meat
Day 6	Full fat soft cheese with celery	Mixed seeds
Day 7	Low carb dessert (see recipes on pages 86 to 90)	Smoked salmon

Step 4: What Can You Eat?

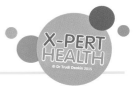

Lunches

Day 1		Homemade cream of mushroom soup
Day 2		Cold meat or fish with salad
Day 3		Low carb pizza (see recipe on page 86 for an example)
Day 4		Avocado and prawns with full fat mayo
Day 5		Frittata with salad
Day 6		Fish or chicken goujons in almond flour with swede French fries
Day 7		Homemade beef or mozzarella burgers with salad

Evening meal

Day 1		Stir-fry with meat, fish or tofu
Day 2		Chicken stuffed with cream cheese and wrapped in bacon
Day 3		Steak with cauliflower mash (see recipe on page 82) and green beans
Day 4		Salmon with rocket and spinach
Day 5		Pork in cream and mushroom sauce served with courgette spaghetti
Day 6		Steak & kidney almond crust pie (see recipe on page 89) with carrot, swede or celeriac fries
Day 7		Chicken curry with cauliflower rice

If you do not want to eat three meals every day, as is common when people follow this dietary approach, you may wish to try intermittent fasting. See pages 48 to 51 for more information.

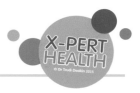

By the time you reach this step you should have a good understanding of what foods you do and do not want to regularly consume. In order to assess if the changes you have made have been sufficient to meet the recommendations for a very low carb dietary approach it is useful to compare the number of portions from each food group that you are consuming with the recommendations for this dietary approach (see page 27).

Assess your diet to see how close it is to what you are aiming for

You can compare your daily intake of food to reference ranges using the Nutrition for Health model. It is simple to do and provides you with immediate feedback about your current dietary approach. To complete this assessment follow the steps below.

1 Consider all the food (meals and snacks) and drinks that you are consuming. You can either complete a food diary (like the one you completed in Step 1) first and then transfer this information to the Nutrition for Health model template on page 33, or you can record it directly on the Nutrition for Health model template.

2 Refer to the 'What is a Portion?' table on page 31 to help work out how many portions you are having of each food, and make a note of this next to each food in the Nutrition for Health model.

Please note that your serving size may be more than one portion, for example a 60g (2 oz.) serving of cheese will provide 2 portions of dairy.

3 When you have finished completing the template add up the number of portions from each food group, and note the number of eating episodes you have each day in the eating frequency box. An example of a completed assessment is shown on page 32.

4 Repeat steps 1 to 3 to assess your diet every day over the next week (using the templates on pages 33 to 39).

5 Compare the number of portions you are having each day with the recommended ranges for a very low carb dietary approach. Use the table on page 40 to help with this, and to identify any goals for change. It is especially important to identify any sources of carbs to help ensure your carb intake has been reduced to less than 50g per day. Use the guidance on pages 22 to 25 to help with this.

Questions to ask yourself about your daily diet – am I consuming:

between 5 and 9 portions of fruit & vegetables? Enough variety? Sufficient non-starchy vegetables and salad and not over consuming fruit?

0 portions of sugary or starchy carbs? Vegetables, fruit, some proteins and some dairy provide carbs. Therefore, to keep carb consumption below 50g, all starchy and sugary foods will need omitting

2 to 3 portions of dairy food? If not, am I obtaining calcium from other sources such as green leafy vegetables, oily fish and nuts?

2 to 4 portions of protein foods? Sufficient variety by including white and oily fish; red meat and poultry; eggs and seafood; pulses, nuts and seeds?

healthy natural fats such as extra virgin olive oil, butter, lard, ghee and coconut oil in preference to processed vegetable oils and spreads made from corn and sunflower?

alcohol in moderation? Not exceeding 2 to 3 units per day and having regular alcohol free days?

real and not **processed foods?**

Step 5: Monitoring Success - What Is A Portion?

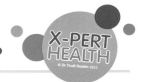

Serving sizes are not always equal to one portion, for example a bowl of cereal can be 3+ portions of carbs! It is therefore important to have an idea of how big a portion actually is.

Food group	Daily portion recommendation and general guidance	What is a portion?
Carbs including starchy & sugary food/drinks	**0 portions** These foods should be omitted when following a very low carb dietary approach, but examples of portion sizes are included for reference Rough guide: a portion of carbs is about one cupped handful	• 2-4 tbs breakfast cereal (20-40g) • 1 slice of bread/toast (40g) • 1 to 2 tbs (40-50g) rice/pasta cooked • 2 boiled/1-2 tbs mashed potato (100-120g) • 1 scoop ice cream/½ packet of crisps • 3 tsp sugar or 1-2 tsp jam/honey (15g)
Fruit & vegetables contain fibre, vitamins and minerals	**5 to 9 portions (at least 400g per day)** Include a variety of salad and other low carb vegetables each day. Only include small portions of low sugar fruit (fresh, frozen, tinned or dried) Rough guide: one portion of veg is about the same size as your fist, and a portion of fruit is about the same size as your palm	• 2-3 tbs vegetables (80g) • Side salad e.g. lettuce, tomato, cucumber • Piece of fresh fruit (80g) • Small handful of berries (80g) • Small cup cherries (80g)
Protein contains essential amino acids	**2 to 4 portions** Choose a variety of protein foods to obtain the essential nutrients. Rough guide: a portion of red meat is roughly the size of a deck of cards or the palm of your hand, and a portion of chicken or fish is roughly the size of your whole hand layed flat	• 85g (3oz) red meat, poultry or oily fish • 120-140g (4-5oz) white fish (unbattered) • 2 eggs • 4 tbs dish based on pulses/lentils/dhal • 60g nuts/2 rounded tbs peanut butter
Dairy contains calcium	**2 to 3 portions** Rough guide: a portion of cheese is about the size of a small matchbox	• 1/3 pint (200ml) cow's milk (or dairy free options, e.g. fortified soya milk or unsweetened almond milk) • Small pot yoghurt/fromage frais (150ml) • 2 tbs cottage cheese (60g) • 30g cheese (1oz)
Fats contains essential fatty acids	**5 to 10 portions** Remember, the type of fat is important (see pages 70 to 73)- avoid processed vegetable oils Rough guide: a portion of fat is about the same size as your thumb	• 2 tsp (14g) natural fat, e.g. butter, lard, coconut oil, suet, dripping, goose fat • 10ml oil (preferably extra virgin olive) • 2 tsp mayonnaise • 10ml oil-based salad dressing • 1 tbs double cream (15-20ml) Note: other fatty foods that might usually be placed in other foods groups, such as nuts or avocado, can be included as a fat portion to help you reach the target of 5-10 portions

tsp = teaspoon, tbs = tablespoon

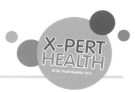

The Nutrition for Health model below is an example of how to complete a dietary self-assessment using the instructions on page 30. Uses the blank templates on page 33 to 39 to complete your own assessment, and compare your results to the recommendations using the table on page 40.

Breakfast
2 egg omelette (made with butter, 10g)
Spinach (3 tbs, 80g)
Mushrooms (2 tbs, 80g)
Cheese (30g)

Evening meal
Beef (85g)
Cauliflower mash (2 tbs, 160g)
(made with butter, 20g)
Mixed veg (4 tbs, 160g)
Butter (for veg, 10g)
Gravy (made with meat juices)

Lunch
Mixed salad (160g)
Extra virgin olive oil (4 tsp, 20g)
Salmon (1 fillet, 85g)

Milk in coffee/tea (200ml, whole milk)

 Frequency of eating: 3

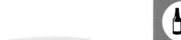 **Alcoholic drinks**
Number of portions: 0

 Fruit & vegetables
Number of portions: 8

 Carbs
Number of portions: 0

1P spinach
1P mushrooms
2P salad
2P cauliflower mash
2P mixed veg

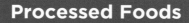 **Processed Foods**

1P butter (omelette)
2P extra-virgin olive oil
2P butter (cauliflower)
1P butter (mix veg)
1P gravy

 Protein
Number of portions: 3

1P eggs (omelette)
1P salmon
1P beef

 Fats
Number of portions: 7

1P cheese
1P milk (whole)

 Dairy
Number of portions: 2

Step 5: Monitoring Success – Dietary Self-Assessment

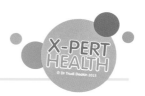

Date: ....

Frequency of eating: ☐

Alcoholic drinks Number of portions: ☐

Carbs Number of portions: ☐

Fruit & vegetables Number of portions: ☐

Processed Foods

Protein Number of portions: ☐

Fats Number of portions: ☐

Dairy Number of portions: ☐

If you find it useful to assess your dietary intake using this method you can download more blank templates from our free online forum; at www.xperthealth.org.uk/forums.

Step 5: Monitoring Success - Dietary Self-Assessment

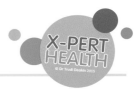

Date: ....

Frequency of eating: ☐

Alcoholic drinks Number of portions: ☐

Carbs Number of portions: ☐

Fruit & vegetables Number of portions: ☐

Processed Foods

Protein Number of portions: ☐

Fats Number of portions: ☐

Dairy Number of portions: ☐

If you find it useful to assess your dietary intake using this method you can download more blank templates from our free online forum; at www.xperthealth.org.uk/forums.

Step 5: Monitoring Success - Dietary Self-Assessment

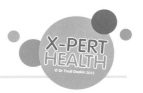

Date: ....

Frequency of eating: ☐

Alcoholic drinks
Number of portions: ☐

Carbs
Number of portions: ☐

Fruit & vegetables
Number of portions: ☐

Processed Foods

Protein
Number of portions: ☐

Fats
Number of portions: ☐

Dairy
Number of portions: ☐

If you find it useful to assess your dietary intake using this method you can download more blank templates from our free online forum; at www.xperthealth.org.uk/forums.

Step 5: Monitoring Success – Dietary Assessment

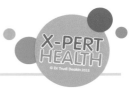

Date: ....

Frequency of eating: ☐

Alcoholic drinks Number of portions: ☐

Carbs Number of portions: ☐

Fruit & vegetables Number of portions: ☐

Processed Foods

Protein Number of portions: ☐

Fats Number of portions: ☐

Dairy Number of portions: ☐

If you find it useful to assess your dietary intake using this method you can download more blank templates from our free online forum; at www.xperthealth.org.uk/forums.

Step 5: Monitoring Success – Dietary Assessment

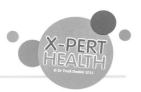

Date: ....

Frequency of eating: ☐

Alcoholic drinks
Number of portions: ☐

Carbs
Number of portions: ☐

Fruit & vegetables
Number of portions: ☐

Processed Foods

Protein
Number of portions: ☐

Fats
Number of portions: ☐

Dairy
Number of portions: ☐

If you find it useful to assess your dietary intake using this method you can download more blank templates from our free online forum; at **www.xperthealth.org.uk/forums**.

Step 5: Monitoring Success - Dietary Assessment

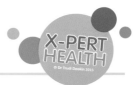

Date: ....

Frequency of eating: ☐

Alcoholic drinks Number of portions: ☐

Carbs Number of portions: ☐

Fruit & vegetables Number of portions: ☐

Processed Foods

Protein Number of portions: ☐

Fats Number of portions: ☐

Dairy Number of portions: ☐

If you find it useful to assess your dietary intake using this method you can download more blank templates from our free online forum; at www.xperthealth.org.uk/forums.

Step 5: Monitoring Success - Dietary Assessment

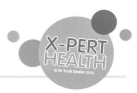

Date: ....

Frequency of eating: ☐

Alcoholic drinks Number of portions: ☐

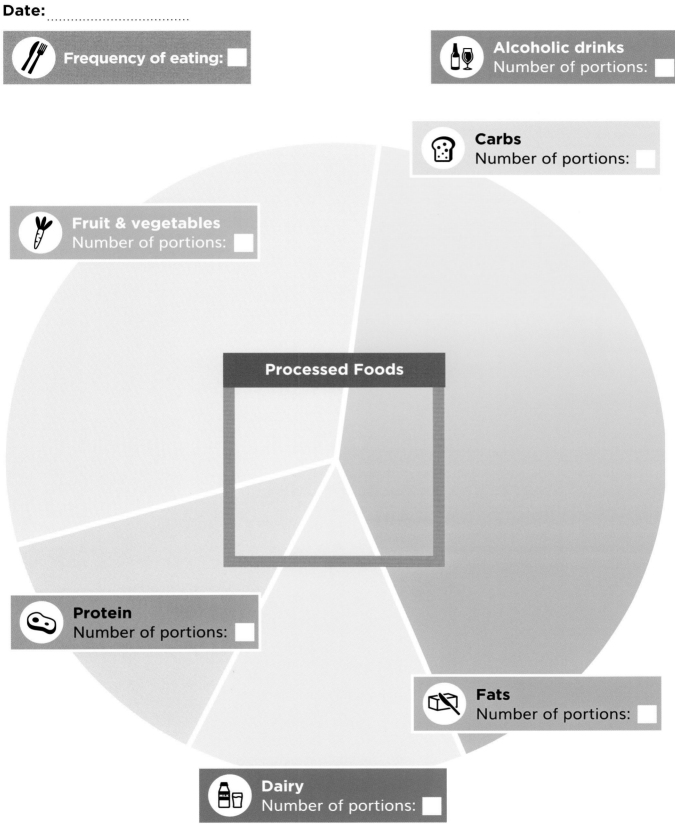

Carbs Number of portions: ☐

Fruit & vegetables Number of portions: ☐

Processed Foods ☐

Protein Number of portions: ☐

Fats Number of portions: ☐

Dairy Number of portions: ☐

If you find it useful to assess your dietary intake using this method you can download more blank templates from our free online forum; at www.xperthealth.org.uk/forums.

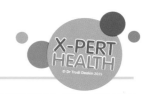

Use the table below to compare your current diet, using the dietary self-assessments from pages 35 to 41, to the recommendations for a very low carb dietary approach.

Reference ranges	Your present diet	Your goals
Carbs		
0 portions per day		
Fruit & vegetables		
5 - 9 portions per day		
Protein		
2 - 4 portions per day		
Dairy		
2 - 3 portions per day		
Fats		
5 - 10 portions per day		
Drinks		
To thirst (1 to 2 litres per day)		
Alcoholic drinks (Maximum 14 units per week, with at least 2 alcohol free days)		
2-3 units per day (maximum)		
Salt (see question 2 on page 42 for info on why it may be necessary to add some salt)		
3-7g per day		
Eating frequency		
No more than 3 eating episodes per day		

Step 6: Maintenance

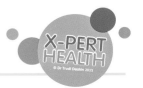

Once you have achieved your health goals* you need to decide what to do next. Be aware that if you reach your goals but return to your previous eating behaviour your health may get worse again. This handbook has encouraged long-term lifestyle changes rather than a short-term 'diet'. Adopting a lifelong dietary approach will enable you to maintain improvements in health. It is therefore essential that you find a dietary approach you enjoy; otherwise it is highly unlikely you will want to, or be able to, stick to it. There are three options:

1 **Remain on a carb-restricted diet**

If you have experienced benefits from restricting carbs you may be happy to remain on a very low carb dietary approach. As long as you are including a variety of 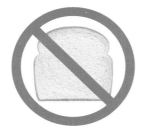 good quality foods you can easily obtain all of the nutrients your body needs whilst following this dietary approach.

2 **Gradually increase carbs to determine your tolerance level**

If you have struggled with the dietary approach and have missed consuming carbs you may wish to experiment with gradually increasing them to see if you are able to consume more without it negatively affecting your health. You could try increasing carbs by 10-20g each week, but cut back again if you can no longer control your weight or any other aspect of your health that is important to you.

If you have benefited from restricting carbs it is recommended that you remain on some form of low carb diet. To do this, try to keep carb consumption below 130g per day and choose slow releasing options (see page 101).

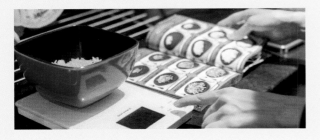

3 **Continue with, or begin, intermittent fasting**

Many people report feeling less hungry when following a very low carb dietary approach. Intermittent fasting can therefore be a suitable option, and can have additional benefits to those many experience when carbs are restricted. If you have experimented with intermittent fasting, whether that be a 5:2 approach or time-restricted eating, and have seen some benefits you may wish to continue with it.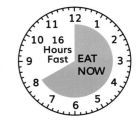

If you haven't experimented with this approach it may be something you wish to try. Easy ways of introducing an element of fasting to your routine can be to simply avoid snacks, or to try time-restricted eating. More information about intermittent fasting, including addressing some of the common myths and misconceptions, can be found on pages 48 to 51.

* If you have not seen the benefits you were hoping for from following this dietary approach it may be worth repeating steps 1 to 5 to see if there are any additional changes you can make. Alternatively you may need to consider if there are any non-dietary factors affecting your health. Things like elevated stress (see page 66), poor sleep (page 67) or not taking part in enough physical activity can significantly affect your health even if you have a healthy dietary approach that suits you.

Frequently Asked Questions

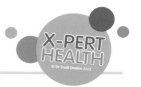

The next few pages address some frequently asked questions to help support you in adopting and sticking to a very low carb dietary approach. There can be an adaptation period when changing your dietary approach so it is essential to understand how you can reduce the risk of any unwanted side effects.

1 **I've heard that a reduced carb diet can lead to constipation, is this true?**

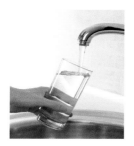

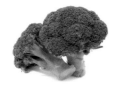

Constipation is usually caused by a lack of dietary fibre, insufficient fluid consumption or a sedentary lifestyle. Therefore, to prevent constipation:

- be as active as possible. Try to be active for 30 minutes or more most days, and break up spells of inactivity by getting up and walking round the room every 20 to 30 minutes

- ensure that you drink enough fluid. It is recommended to consume 1 to 2 litres per day. If your urine is light coloured this is an indication that you are hydrated

- consume plenty of fibre. The fibre recommendation in the UK for adults is 30g per day. You can increase your fibre intake by having 5 to 9 portions of low carb fruit & vegetables each day, although fibre intake should be increased gradually to prevent unwanted side effects, e.g. bloating. Additional fibre can be obtained by consuming low carb high fibre foods (see pages 102 and 103)

2 **I feel shaky and hungry - why is this?**

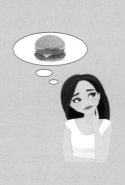

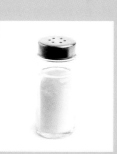

If you are insulin resistant you will have been releasing extra insulin to help control blood glucose levels. Now that you have reduced your intake of carbs it may take a little time for your pancreas to recognise that you do not require the additional insulin any more. The high concentration of insulin in your blood may result in your blood glucose levels dropping to a lower level than your body is used to. Don't worry though, it is very unlikely that they will drop to a level that is dangerous **unless you are taking certain medication; see question 3.** For a few days, until your body has adjusted to your lower blood glucose levels, you may experience mild hypoglycaemia ("hypo") symptoms such as shakiness, hunger and headaches. Stick with it and these symptoms will pass. Do not feel tempted to have a sugary drink or snack as this will once again trigger the release of insulin, which will make the problem worse. It may help relieve the symptoms if you have a drink such as coffee, tea or water.

You may also need to consume more salt. When following a very low carb dietary approach people tend to consume fewer processed foods, reducing their salt intake, and have lower insulin levels, which leads to more sodium (a component of salt) being excreted from the body. This combination of factors can lead to low sodium levels, which can cause dizziness. Adding salt to food, to taste, can address this.

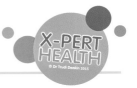

3 Will a very low carb lifestyle affect the medication I take?

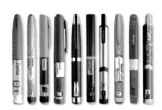

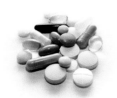

If you have diabetes and are prescribed a type of medication called sulphonylureas, or you are injecting insulin, **you will need to discuss a reduction or change in your medication before you start restricting carbs.** Examples of sulphonylureas are Gliclazide (Diamicron), Glipizide (Minodiab), Glimepiride (Amaryl), Glibenclamide and Tolbutamide. Sulphonylureas work by stimulating cells in the pancreas to make more insulin. If you reduce your intake of carbs without adjusting doses of this medication and/or insulin it is likely that blood glucose levels will drop too low and you will experience hypoglycemia ("hypos"). Severe hypos need to be treated with glucose immediately to prevent the brain being starved of glucose, and there is a risk of becoming unconscious.

Conditions such as heartburn and high blood pressure have also been shown to improve with a reduced carb lifestyle and you may be able to reduce or even omit medication as a result. **Book an appointment with your doctor to review your health results and medication.**

4 I am not losing weight as quickly as I would like. Why is this?

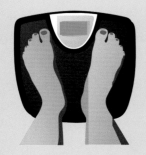

If you are trying to lose weight but are not meeting your goals you will naturally be disappointed. It may be worth repeating steps 1 to 4 in this handbook, focusing on whether you have reduced your carb intake sufficiently and whether you are eating too frequently.

Possible reasons for not achieving weight loss goals include consuming too many carbs and eating when you are not hungry (see pages 62 to 65 for more on this). A reduced carb lifestyle tends to be more satisfying and, although you don't need to count calories, if you override your appetite and eat to excess you can still gain weight. When people learn to read their appetite they often find they reduce the number of meals and snacks they consume naturally.

Although fats tend to be more filling some fatty foods, such as nuts and cheese, are still easily overconsumed. This can prevent weight loss. If you have restricted carbs but are still struggling to manage your weight it may be that you would benefit from reducing the number of fat portions you consume. Remember, some of the "high fat" part of this dietary approach can come from your stored body fat rather than from fat in your diet.

Ensure that your weight loss goals are realistic. Typically it is realistic and safe to achieve 0.5kg to 1kg weight loss per week, although some individuals will achieve more or less than this.

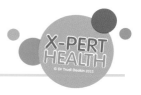
5 **Is it OK to follow a reduced carb dietary approach if I have a medical condition such as diabetes or kidney disease?**

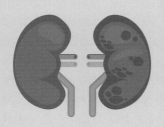

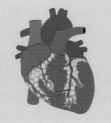

If you have a medical condition it is wise to check with your healthcare team before adopting a very low carb lifestyle. However, reducing carbs has been shown to be effective for lowering blood glucose and weight in some people with type 1 or type 2 diabetes and so can be a good option for many people. Some medications will need to be reduced before adopting this approach though (see question 3).

Some people are concerned about the impact of protein on the kidneys. This diet is not high protein anyway, but if you are healthy with no kidney disease eating extra protein will not cause harm. However, if you have a history of kidney disease you may need to fill up on healthy fats rather that eating larger protein portions.

6 **Is this dietary approach expensive?**

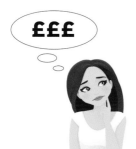

You may worry that purchasing real, unprocessed foods to meet the guidance for this dietary approach will be expensive. Although some of the individual ingredients recommended can cost more there are a number of factors that can compensate for this, and you may even reduce your overall food spend:

- Many people reduce snacks and their frequency of eating on this dietary approach (see pages 48 to 51). If you are eating less often you won't need to buy as much food!

- Buying the basic ingredients to cook from scratch can be cheaper than relying on ready meals and convenience meals

- You can purchase popular ingredients in bulk, which is cheaper than purchasing smaller quantities. Some commonly used ingredients, for example sweeteners or ground almonds, have long shelf lives so are suitable for bulk buying

- Other staple foods, such as eggs and tinned oily fish, are cheap and highly nutritious

- You can purchase vegetables and low sugar fruits frozen, which can reduce waste and help save money

- Although fatty foods with higher protein content, such as meat, fish and cheese, can be more expensive there are cheaper fatty options - such as lard and dripping - that can be used for cooking and will help fill you up

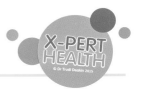

7 **What about weight loss supplements, will they help me to lose weight?**

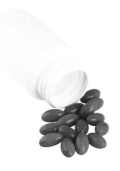

Supplements are often marketed as having huge benefits in relation to health and weight loss. Although there is some evidence that certain supplements may have beneficial effects there is no strong and consistent evidence that any particular supplement should be recommended. For this reason we have not included any specific examples in this handbook. More research is needed, but there is no reason you cannot meet all of your health goals by eating a real food diet. If you are currently taking any supplements, and you feel they are benefiting you, there is no reason why you should stop taking them. You can ask any questions you have about specific supplements using our free online forum, accessible at www.xperthealth.org.uk/forums.

8 **Does a low carb dietary approach cause bad breath?**

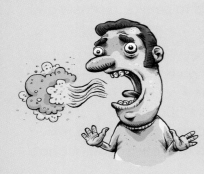

Reducing carb intake results in more fat being used for energy, generating ketones (see page 13). One type of ketone, acetone, tends to be excreted in urine and in the breath. This can cause bad breath. The description of the smell varies but it is often described as "fruity" or like the smell of pear drops. The good news is that "keto-breath" usually doesn't last for long. Most people find it dies down after a few weeks as they adapt to using the ketones for energy. However, there are things you can do to minimise the impact of "keto-breath" in the meantime:

- Drink more water
- Use natural breath fresheners such as mint, parsley, cloves, cinnamon and fennel seeds
- Try breath capsules, e.g. Mint Asure. These are usually made from parsley oil
- Try sugar-free mints or gum

9 **I feel really tired, is this normal?**

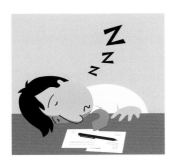

Whilst your body is adapting to using fat as its preferred fuel rather than carbs you may feel a little more tired than usual. This is because your body will not be used to relying on fat and ketones for most of its energy. However, this will be short-lived and after a week or two you will probably find that your energy levels improve considerably. Many people even report feeling much more energetic than they did before. This is because we have a vast amount of fat stored in our body, so if we can access it efficiently it can provide a constant supply of energy.

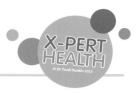

10 Is the dietary approach nutritionally complete or do I need to take nutritional supplements?

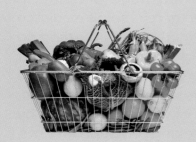

Critics of the reduced carb lifestyle often state that it will result in being deficient in vitamin C and certain B vitamins. However, as long as you are eating a good variety of food, e.g. leafy green vegetables, nuts and berries, natural fats (such as butter, lard, olive oil, coconut oil), meats, poultry, and fish, you will probably be consuming MORE vitamins and minerals than you did on your previous diet! There is not usually any need for supplements, although some people may have to add some salt to their food (as discussed in question 2, on page 42). Many of the carb containing foods that you will be omitting are not very nutrient dense.

11 Is it possible to be gluten/wheat/lactose free on a very low carb dietary approach?

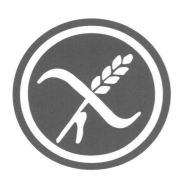

Absolutely, this can be a good option for people with coeliac disease (a lifelong autoimmune disease caused by intolerance to gluten), dermatitis herpetiformis (a skin condition linked to coeliac disease) and intolerances to wheat and lactose.

Gluten is a protein found in wheat, rye and barley; and a similar protein is found in oats. It is therefore easy to follow a very low carb dietary approach that is gluten and wheat-free as these carb-rich grains are omitted when carbs are restricted to less than 50g per day anyway. Flour substitutes such as ground almonds, coconut and golden milled flaxseed that do not contain gluten can be used to make bread, scones, pastry, cakes and biscuits if desired.

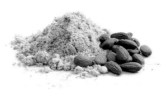

Lactose intolerance is a common digestive problem where the body is unable to digest lactose, a type of sugar mainly found in dairy products. A major source of lactose is milk (cow, goat and sheep) and products made from milk such as butter, cream, ice cream, cream cheese and milk chocolate. Some dairy products however, such as hard cheese, double cream and yogurt, contain lower levels of lactose than milk. Depending on how severe your lactose intolerance is you may need to reduce the amount of milk in your diet or avoid it entirely. This can be easily done on a very low carb dietary approach, because:

- breakfast cereals, which are usually consumed with milk, are omitted
- double cream contains less lactose and can replace milk in drinks and sauces
- calcium requirements can be achieved from eating full fat yogurt and hard cheese, or through consuming certain vegetables
- processed food with hidden sources of milk/milk products are reduced or omitted
- you can purchase unsweetened milk made from soya, almonds, hazelnuts and coconut

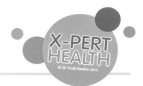

12 Is this not just another fad diet?

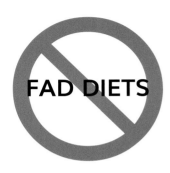

The majority of diets are marketed purely as a short-term weight loss solution, focused solely on reducing the intake of calories. However, these tend to result in weight regain due to a reduction in basal metabolic rate (BMR); i.e. the body reduces the amount of energy it uses because it thinks it is being deprived. These diets do not consider the hormones that drive appetite and fat storage.

A very low carb dietary approach is not a fad diet, it is a style of eating that can be adopted for life. It can support you in improving your health, allow you to obtain and maintain a healthy body weight, and can also help prevent and/or treat a whole host of other conditions (see pages 10 to 12).

This approach is backed by science, with its primary aim being to tackle high insulin levels and insulin resistance. Carbs are the main stimulator of insulin and insulin is the main stimulator of insulin resistance. Therefore, restricting carbs lowers insulin levels and reduces insulin resistance. This can help you to use the fat stored in your body as an energy source, which will help you to lose weight. This ability to access stored fat also means the body does not feel like it is being deprived, preventing the reduction in BMR seen with the calorie restricted diets many people try.

However, you will only succeed as long as you follow the dietary approach. If you revert to your previous style of eating, it is likely that many of the benefits you might see will be reversed.

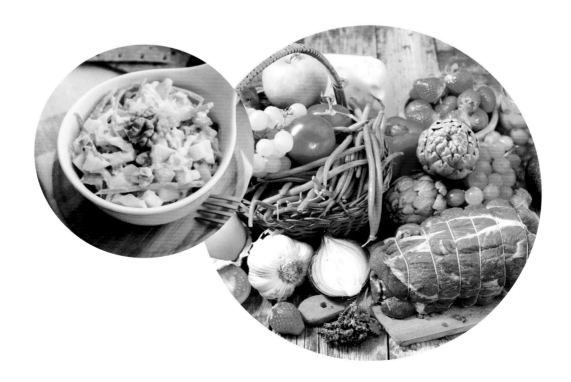

Intermittent Fasting

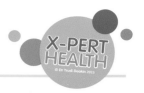

As mentioned previously, it is common for those following a very low carb dietary approach to feel less hungry. Intermittent fasting is therefore often practiced alongside this dietary approach, and it can have some additional benefits.

What is intermittent fasting?

Intermittent fasting is an eating pattern where you cycle between periods of eating and fasting. There are several different intermittent fasting methods, all of which split the day or week into eating periods and fasting periods. The options are vast and can be changed from week to week to fit in with your schedule.

Two examples discussed below are the 5:2 diet and time-restricted eating:

The 5:2 diet

This is a fasting diet plan that limits calorie intake for 2 days per week. The two days of fasting require keeping dietary intake below a set number of calories: 500 for women or 600 for men.

It doesn't have to be a true 'fast' as the name implies. You don't have to go for two days without eating anything, but you can do if you would like to. Also, you do not have to fast on two consecutive days. You can choose the two most convenient days in the week and they can be different days each week if you wish.

There are other approaches similar to this, with more fasting days, such as fasting for 4 days and eating for 3, or fewer fasts, such as fasting for 1 day and eating for 6.

Time-restricted eating

In this approach you select an eating window, usually between four hours (such as from 2pm to 6pm) and eight hours (such as from 11am to 7pm), and only eat during these times. This is commonly performed simply by not having breakfast, which results in an extended fast between the previous evening's meal and lunch (or dinner if a longer fast is desired). Time-restricted eating can be undertaken every day or just on certain days of the week.

Initially people may find it difficult to miss an entire meal, but often report that it becomes easier over time. Some people may choose to do an extended 24 hour fast, for example from their evening meal on a Monday until their evening meal on Tuesday.

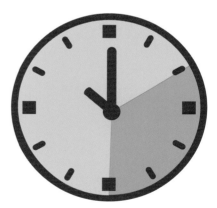

What are the benefits?

The main reason for following a fasting diet is to further reduce insulin levels and insulin resistance. Fasting for extended periods allows our insulin levels to drop, resulting in periods where we are able to use our body's fat stores as energy. Fasting can therefore amplify the impact of a low carb dietary approach and can be beneficial for weight loss and for reducing insulin resistance.

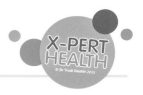

The graph below demonstrates that having frequent meals and snacks increases insulin levels and reduces the amount of time that the body is able to burn fat for energy.

Three meals a day with regular snacking

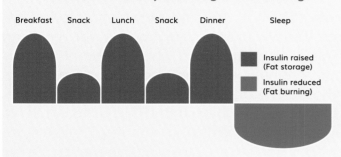

If someone is able to omit snacks and just consume three regular meals there is more time over a 24 hour period where they are able to burn their stored body fat for energy.

Three meals a day

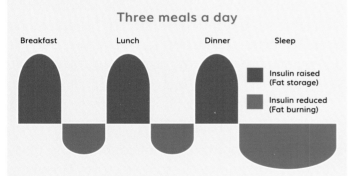

Whereas, consuming just 1 or 2 meals per day vastly increases the fat burning opportunity.

Example of following an intermittent fasting (time restricted eating) protocol

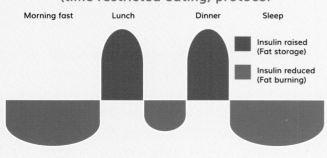

What are the negatives?

There are several myths and misconceptions surrounding fasting which may result in you being wary about trying it. But as long as the food you are eating when you break your fast is nutritionally dense, real food (see page 74) there are not any concerns associated with intermittent fasting. In fact, this is a more natural pattern of eating as humans did not evolve eating three meals per day.

It is however important to note that if you are prescribed any medication(s) you should consult with your GP/healthcare team before fasting, especially if you have certain conditions, such as diabetes, where medication may cause blood glucose levels to drop (see page 43).

Some of the myths related to intermittent fasting are addressed on pages 50 and 51. This may help to ease any concerns you have around fasting.

Although it is beyond the scope of this handbook to discuss intermittent fasting in detail there is lots of support available for people who are interested. The following links may be useful for more information:

www.xperthealth.org.uk/Dietary-Approaches

www.healthline.com/nutrition/intermittent-fasting-guide

www.dietdoctor.com/?s=intermittent+fasting

idmprogram.com/tag/fasting/

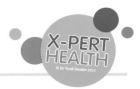

Intermittent fasting can be an excellent option for many people to help them improve their health. Unfortunately however there are a number of myths that lead to people being reluctant to practice it. A number of these myths are addressed over the next two pages.

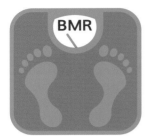

If you fast you will slow your metabolism because you need to eat regular meals and snacks to keep your metabolic rate high

Your basal metabolic rate (BMR) is the rate at which calories are burned at rest. Over time this will drop if your body is not receiving the energy it requires. This is often the case when someone adopts a reduced calorie diet but continues to graze throughout the day, as insulin levels remain high and the body will be in fat storage mode. Insufficient energy is available to the body so BMR drops to conserve energy. This does not happen whilst fasting as the insulin levels are low and fat stored in the body can start to be used for energy. Plenty of energy is therefore available, so the body doesn't need to go into "starvation mode" and slow your metabolism.

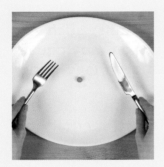

Fasting is just starving yourself

Fasting is a voluntary action to avoid food for a pre-selected period of time. The body doesn't go into starvation mode because it is receiving energy from your fat stores. Starvation is different. True starvation is where food is no longer available for extended periods of time, leading to malnourishment, whereas dietary starvation is where the body is in fat storage mode and *perceives* that energy is no longer available because it cannot access it.

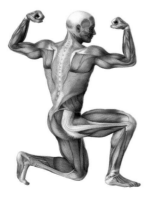

Fasting makes your body break down muscle

No permanent muscle loss occurs with intermittent fasting. The body will always use glucose and fat for energy before it starts breaking down muscle, whilst fasting also increases levels of a growth hormone that protects muscle from being used for energy. Intermittent fasting may even be good for muscle regeneration, as it promotes a process called autophagy. Autophagy is where the body clears out old proteins so they can be replaced with new ones, which are of a higher quality and are less likely to be damaged.

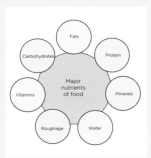

Fasting will deprive you of some essential nutrients

As long as the foods you consume in the non-fasting periods are of sufficient quality there is no reason why all of the essential nutrients your body requires cannot be obtained when following this dietary approach. Studies looking at intermittent fasting have found no evidence of malnourishment or nutrient deficiencies. When your body breaks down its fat stores for energy stored nutrients can be re-used.

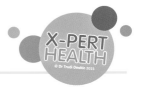

Fasting just makes you hungry all the time and skipping meals makes you eat more at the next meal

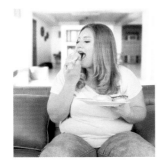

Studies have shown that missing a meal may result in a slight increase in energy intake at the next meal, but the total energy consumed will still likely be much less than if you had eaten both meals.

Eating is either psychologically based (habit, boredom, stress or other emotions; see pages 63 to 65) or mediated through hunger hormones (see below). Fasting decreases hunger hormones and increases satiety (fullness). You may feel hungry at first but this will mostly be for psychological reasons. Once established on an intermittent fasting regime most people report reduced hunger.

Breakfast is the most important meal of the day

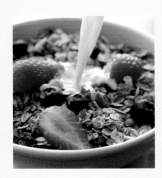

Many people omit breakfast when intermittent fasting as it is a practical way to achieve an extended fasting period, but conventional wisdom says that breakfast is the most important meal of the day. This is not true however. Upon waking the body's internal clock increases adrenaline, growth hormone and cortisol*. These stimulate your body to release energy to start your day. Therefore, consuming food first thing in the morning is not essential. If you enjoy breakfast but still wish to practice some form of intermittent fasting you can always omit a different meal. One size doesn't fit all and so it is important to find an approach that works for you.

* having elevated cortisol levels is not a problem when it is in short bursts, but being stressed (see page 66) can result in elevated levels for prolonged periods, which can be bad for us (see pages 68 and 69)

Fasting and hormones

Fasting helps you to lose weight because it decreases levels of hormones that make you feel hungry and store fat, and increases levels of hormones that make you feel full.

These weight-promoting hormones are decreased:

Insulin – all foods can increase insulin (some more than others). Therefore fasting reduces insulin levels and can also help the insulin you do have to work better.

Ghrelin – is released from the stomach and tells your brain that you are hungry. Studies have shown that fasting decreases levels, reducing your appetite.

These hormones that support weight loss are increased:

Leptin and PYY – help you to feel full, i.e. create satiety. Fasting increases levels, reducing your appetite and making you less inclined to overeat when you break the fast.

Growth hormone – has a vital role in cell turnover, growth and maintaining healthy tissues. It protects muscle mass and increases the availability of fat for fuel.

Adrenaline – is often known for preparing the body for fight or flight, i.e. to deal with danger. However, adrenaline levels can also be raised during non-stressful events such as fasting, which increases metabolism and can therefore have a positive effect.

Reading And Understanding Food Labels

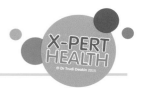

Nutrition labels provide a lot of useful information, but food packaging is ultimately designed to try and influence your decisions. The amount of information presented can be overwhelming, and the claims manufacturers make about their products can be misleading. This section provides you with useful advice regarding which parts of this information can help you make good decisions, and which parts you're best ignoring!

1. The ingredients list

INGREDIENTS: SUGAR, ENRICHED BLEACHED FLOUR (WHEAT FLOUR, NIACIN, REDUCED IRON, THIAMIN MONONITRATE, RIBOFLAVIN, FOLIC ACID), SEMI-SWEET CHOCOLATE CHIPS (SUGAR, CHOCOLATE LIQUOR, COCOA BUTTER, SOY LECITHIN [EMULSIFIER], VANILLA), COCOA (PROCESSED WITH ALKALI), CANOLA OR SOYBEAN OIL, BITTERSWEET CHOCOLATE CHIPS (CHOCOLATE LIQUOR, SUGAR, COCOA BUTTER, MILK FAT, SOY LECITHIN [EMULSIFIER], VANILLA), MILK CHOCOLATE CHIPS (SUGAR, WHOLE MILK POWDER, CHOCOLATE LIQUOR, COCOA BUTTER, SOY LECITHIN [EMULSIFIER], VANILLA), SALT, ARTIFICIAL FLAVOR, SODIUM BICARBONATE.

All ingredients in the product have to be listed in order of the greatest weight. Therefore, in the example above the ingredient with the highest content is 'sugar' and the lowest content 'sodium bicarbonate'.

The length of the list can also indicate how processed the food item is. A longer ingredients list is more likely to suggest that the food has been highly processed, whereas a minimally processed food is likely to have a much shorter ingredients list (many natural, healthy foods don't have an ingredients list at all).

Allergy and intolerance information can also often be found within the ingredients list.

Individual ingredients can be listed under different names, for example, added sugars may be listed as sugar, sucrose, glucose, glucose syrup, invert syrup, maltose, fructose, lactose etc. When listed separately, it can give the impression that there is less added sugar in the product. For more specific details you should check the nutritional information table.

2. The nutritional information table

As a guide, we recommend this product provides: NUTRITION			4 servings
Typical values (microwaved)	Per 100g	Per pot	Reference Intake
Energy	437kJ	874kJ	8400kJ
	104kcal	207kcal	2000kcal
Fat	0.4g	0.8g	70g
of which saturates	0.1g	0.2g	20g
Carbohydrate	17.9g	35.8g	260g
of which sugars	5.7g	11.4g	90g
Fibre	5.2g	10.4g	24g
Protein	4.5g	9.0g	50g
Salt	0.7g	1.4g	6g
STORAGE			
Store in a cool, dry place.			

A table normally displayed at the back of the package with the amount of the main nutrients in that food. Some products will provide more information than others; for example, some may include nutrients per serving or the type of fat.

Many products display nutritional information per 100g and per serving. The amount per serving is useful if you eat the recommended serving size. The 'per 100g' allows easier comparison with different products/brands. It also helps you identify whether a food or drink contains 'a lot' or 'a little' energy (calories), carbs, protein, fat and fibre.

Information about the amount of vitamins and minerals in the product are also sometimes provided in this table, particularly for salt. If the food is a good source of a particular nutrient; for example, vitamin C, calcium or iron, it is more likely to be included in the nutritional information table, although this information isn't always available. This table usually includes reference intake values too.

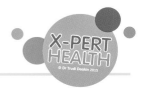

3. Reference intake (RI) labelling

Calories	2000kcal
Total fat	70g
Saturates	20g
Total carbs	260g
Sugars	90g
Protein	50g
Salt	6g

Reference Intakes, previously known as Guideline Daily Amounts (GDAs), provide guidance about the appropriate amount of particular nutrients and energy someone following a low fat diet requires. It is usually displayed on the front of food packaging and/or in the nutritional information table. It states the amount of calories, fat, saturated fat, sugar and salt that can be found in a serving. It also presents what proportion (%) of the RI there is in a serving.

Each pie contains

Energy 975KJ 232kcal	Fat 8.4g	Saturates 2.9g	Sugars 19.2g	Salt 0.2g
12%	12%	15%	21%	3%

RIs are a reference for a healthy adult and are not intended as targets because we all have individual requirements. RIs on food packaging will not be helpful for you when adopting a very low carb dietary approach. Instead, as much as possible, make sure that food contains less than 10g carbs per 100g and you have a diet of sufficient quality to meet your other nutrient requirements.

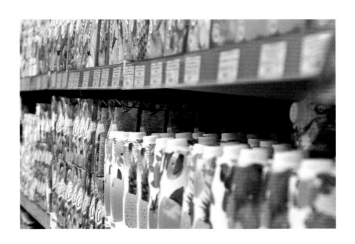

4. Traffic light labelling

The traffic light labelling system has been developed to support adoption of a low fat diet. It assists the consumer in understanding the amount of fat, saturated fat, sugar and salt a product contains and how these compare to government recommendations. It also allows people to compare different products and brands. It doesn't consider the quality of food however, so a product can have red lights for fat and saturated fat despite being a healthy, natural food that would be a good choice for any dietary approach.

As with RIs, traffic light labelling will not help you to adopt a very low carb dietary approach. Therefore, ignore the traffic light colour coding when you are adopting this dietary approach! Concentrate on the ingredients list and nutritional information table instead.

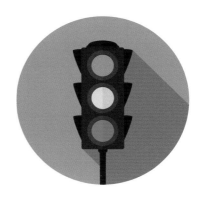

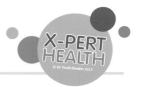

Confused?

There is a lot of information on food labelling that can make it difficult to decide which foods are suitable for your new dietary approach. The information on the previous two pages should help with this, and some additional factors to consider include:

• The RI and Traffic Light labelling systems on the front of packages do not include total carbs, and therefore are not as helpful for people who wish to monitor carb intake. To obtain that information the consumer will have to read the nutritional table which is normally found on the back of the package. For example, the sample nutritional table (below) for mackerel fillets informs the consumer that there is only a trace of carbs per 100g.

• Some foods have a red traffic light but may be beneficial for health. For example: oily fish has a red light for total fat and saturated fat (again, see the image below), but it provides an excellent source of nutrition with good quality protein and omega-3 fats that are health-promoting. Dairy products are real foods and their consumption is important to ensure adequate intake of vitamins and minerals, e.g. calcium; but they may display an amber or red light for sugar, total fat and saturated fat. Nuts will display a red traffic light for total fat and saturated fat, but unprocessed nuts are an excellent source of fibre, healthy fats, vitamins and minerals. Therefore, do not be fearful of purchasing wholesome natural foods which have been colour-coded amber or red.

• Some food packaging will also contain claims about the nutritional content of the product. These can be confusing, and so the table on the following page has been provided to help you identify what these claims actually mean.

Nutrition		Reference Intake	
Typical Values	per 100g	Average adult	per portion
Energy value	1340 kJ	8400 kJ	17%
(kcal	325 kcal)	2000 kcal	
Fat	27.8 g	70 g	40%
(of which Saturates	8.3 g)	20 g	42%
Carbohydrate	Trace g	260 g	<1%
(of which sugars	Trace g)	90 g	<1%
Fibre	Trace g		
Protein	18.2 g	50 g	37%
Salt	1.8 g	6 g	30%
Reference intake of an average adult (8400kJ/2000kcal)			
Serves 2			

Nutritional Claims

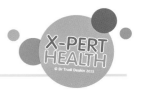

Nutritional claims	What do they mean?
Fat free/ sugar free	Contains very small amounts of fat or sugar (less than 0.5g per 100g). Sugar free foods may be suitable for this dietary approach, as long as they don't contain lots of carbs, but it is not necessary to choose fat free foods*
Reduced fat/ sugar	Contains at least 30% less fat/sugar than its regular comparable product. It is not necessary to reduce fat on this dietary approach*, but it is important to be aware that a reduced sugar food can still contain a lot of sugar and so may not be suitable for this dietary approach. Reduced sugar jam, for example, can still have more than 40g sugar per 100g!
No added sugar	No sugar has been added to the product. When looking at a label it may still show the sugar content to be high, but this will be natural sugars (e.g. fructose in fruit juice). All sugars, whether natural or added, can raise blood glucose levels and have other negative health effects however. These foods may not be suitable for this dietary approach, as they can still contain a lot of carbs.
Low salt	Contains no more than 0.3g salt per 100g product. Reducing salt has only been shown to be beneficial for individuals with hypertension who already consume a lot of salt. When carb intake is significantly reduced it may even be necessary to increase salt intake, as you will typically be consuming less and the reduction in insulin levels can lead to you losing more from the body in the urine. This nutritional claim is therefore not relevant when following this dietary approach.
High fibre	Contains at least 6g fibre per 100g product, or at least 3g per 100kcal. Fibre has many health benefits, so trying to include some products with high fibre content is advisable. Aim to consume 20 to 30g per day. See pages 102 and 103 for more information about fibre and the foods that are good sources of it.
High protein	At least 20% of the calories in the product are from protein. It is recommended to consume 2 to 4 portions of good quality protein each day, but it is better to meet your protein requirements from real foods rather than packaged or processed foods that might carry this claim.

* Processed foods that are high in fat should still be avoided. See page 26 and pages 70 to 73 for more information about different fats and the foods that contain them

Top 10 Food Shopping Tips

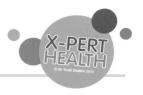

As well as possible difficulties in understanding the information on food labels there are a number of other challenges we face when food shopping. To help minimise these we have included 10 tips to help you out!

Tip	Specific advice for a very low carb lifestyle

① Examine the ingredients list

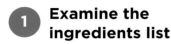

INGREDIENTS: SUGAR, ENRICHED BLEACHED FLOUR (WHEAT FLOUR, NIACIN, REDUCED IRON, THIAMIN MONONITRATE, RIBOFLAVIN, FOLIC ACID), SEMI-SWEET CHOCOLATE CHIPS (SUGAR, CHOCOLATE LIQUOR, COCOA BUTTER, SOY LECITHIN [EMULSIFIER], VANILLA), COCOA (PROCESSED WITH ALKALI), CANOLA OR SOYBEAN OIL, BITTERSWEET CHOCOLATE CHIPS (CHOCOLATE LIQUOR, SUGAR, COCOA BUTTER, MILK FAT, SOY LECITHIN [EMULSIFIER], VANILLA), MILK CHOCOLATE CHIPS (SUGAR, WHOLE MILK POWDER, CHOCOLATE LIQUOR, COCOA BUTTER, SOY LECITHIN [EMULSIFIER], VANILLA), SALT, ARTIFICIAL FLAVOR, SODIUM BICARBONATE.

The ingredients list can provide you with some useful information (see page 52). For this dietary approach you should be choosing products which mainly list fat, protein or fibre based ingredients; and avoiding foods which contain starches or sugars at the top of the ingredients list. You should also mostly be choosing real foods which contain a minimal number of ingredients.

② Ignore the traffic light labelling system

Traffic light labelling can be misleading (see page 53). Do not be fearful of purchasing wholesome, natural foods which have been colour-coded amber or red for fat and salt. Foods that are often flagged as red, suggesting a "less healthy choice", include oily fish, nuts and full-fat dairy products. This is incorrect as these foods are in fact health promoting, and are good choices when following a very low carb dietary approach.

③ Ignore the reference intakes but consider the nutritional table

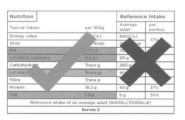

Reference intakes (see page 53) are not useful if you are following a very low carb or intermittent fasting dietary approach. Ignore them!

The nutritional information table (see page 52) is useful however as it will be able to guide you to choose foods that will support your chosen dietary approach. For example, a food that is less than 10g per 100g of carbs may be suitable for a very low carb dietary approach.

④ Avoid the end of aisles

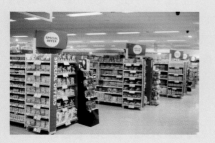

In food stores, particularly large 'superstores', the end of aisles often feature special offers. Whilst being financially tempting these special offers are often highly processed foods which contain a lot of refined carbs and/or processed fats. These foods tend to be detrimental to health and rarely support a reduced carb or intermittent fasting dietary approach.

To avoid temptation try to just ignore the banners and promotional material advertising 'special offers'!

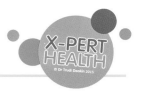

Tip	Specific advice for a very low carb lifestyle

5 **Plan meals and make a list**

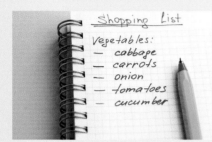

Organisation is key when adopting a new dietary approach. Plan the meals for the week ahead and write down the ingredients on a shopping list. One common mistake is to go shopping and purchase favourite snack foods or familiar convenience meals. These are unlikely to support your new dietary approach.

Purchasing natural ingredients based on meals you are going to make from scratch will reduce your intake of processed foods. If processed, unhealthy foods are not on your list and you do not buy them, you will not eat them! Writing a shopping list will help to reduce temptation and may even reduce how much you spend on your weekly shop!

6 **Never go food shopping when hungry**

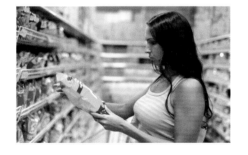

Where possible do not go food shopping when you are hungry. Shopping when you are hungry may increase the likelihood of you making impulse purchases and choosing less healthy choices that do not support your new dietary approach.

Avoiding going shopping when you are hungry can also help to prevent you spending more money than you intended.

7 **Go for diversity**

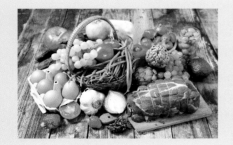

A varied diet, which includes many different types of real foods, can improve your gut health. A diverse real food diet will also increase your intake of vitamins, minerals and fibre.

Purchasing real ingredients will support you in cooking meals from scratch, and this frequently adds flavour and essential nutrients to your meals as well as filling you up for longer than highly processed foods will.

Aim to have a shopping basket full of colourful products such as: fresh vegetables, salad ingredients and low sugar fruits, healthy fats, high quality proteins and full fat dairy products. Avoid foods high in sugar and processed fats such as ready meals, confectionary, vegetable oils, low fat dairy, processed meats and baked goods.

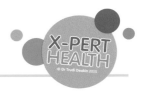

Tip	Specific advice for a very low carb lifestyle

8 **Consider the 'Foods For Fullness'**

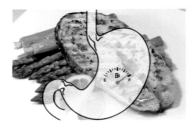

Some foods are really good at "filling you up", whereas others are not. When shopping try to choose foods that you know will fill you up more and avoid foods that won't. As a simple rule of thumb, vegetables (largely because of their fibre content, see pages 102 and 103) and unprocessed, high-quality proteins and fats- such as eggs, fish (particularly oily), grass fed meats, and cheese-offer a greater fullness factor than refined and processed foods.

9 **Don't shop alone**

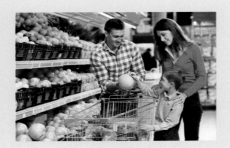

Some people find food shopping really boring and therefore may purchase familiar and tempting foods thinking that they will alleviate the boredom and make the shopping experience more enjoyable. They may also feel that purchasing familiar foods will save time rather than seeking out new products that support their new dietary approach.

Try to think of another way to make the shopping trip more enjoyable such as asking a friend, family member or partner to go shopping with you; or perhaps organise something afterwards to look forward to.

10 **Do a weekly food shop**

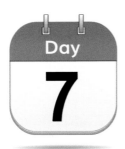

Try to aim for just one large food shop each week to accommodate all your needs. When people break down their food shopping into several 'top-up' shops, less healthy choices may be made as you are increasing the number of times that you may be tempted to purchase familiar favourite foods that you have missed since starting on your new dietary approach.

Doing a weekly shop, if planned well, is often a more time and cost efficient way to purchase food.

If you are interested in trying some of the carb swaps or in making some of the reduced carb recipes, see pages 82 to 90, you may find it useful to purchase some of the staple ingredients in bulk at a reduced fee; e.g. ground almonds, golden milled flaxseed and xylitol/erythritol. These can be obtained from Amazon (**www.amazon. co.uk**), for example, and there are also online shops that specialise in reduced carb products. Some of these are listed on page 121.

Top 10 Dining Out Tips

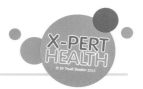

Many people avoid dining out when adopting a new dietary approach, but this is unnecessary. If you are going to stick to your new dietary approach it is essential that you enjoy it, and being able to dine out can be an important part of that. Here are some top tips to help you enjoy dining out whilst adopting a very low carb dietary approach.

Tip

Why?

1 **Do not be afraid of dining out!**

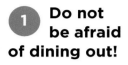

Dining out is a great way to enjoy good food with family and friends.

Eating meals out should be a relaxing and enjoyable experience that can help to reduce the stress of everyday life. Reducing stress levels can assist in weight loss as it will reduce stress hormone levels (see pages 66 to 69).

2 **Consider the 'Foods For Fullness'**

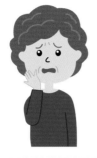

Don't be in a rush to order your meal. Consider the different ingredients in each dish, as this will help you choose a meal that supports your dietary approach and help to keep you full for the longest period of time. Foods containing protein, fats and soluble fibre will help you feel full.

3 **Think what foods will drive up your insulin levels**

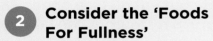
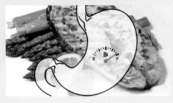

If you see a meal that would be suitable for a very low carb dietary approach but it is served with carbs (such as potato, fries, rice, pasta or bread) don't be afraid to ask to swap for low carb substitutes such as vegetables or salad. Also remember that as you are reducing the carbs, you need to increase fat consumption. So you may want to ask for butter, olive oil or mayonnaise to add to the swaps to prevent you going hungry!

4 **Be adventurous when ordering**

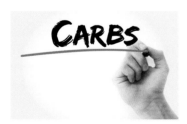
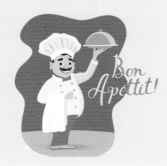

Try experimenting and order something that you haven't tried before. If you don't understand some of the items on the menu, ask! Waiters should be able to explain what the dish is and the ingredients it contains. With the popularity of alternative dietary approaches chefs are creating lots of new and exciting recipes using healthier ingredients such as bolognese with courgette spaghetti ("courgetti") rather than pasta. Therefore restaurants are great places to try new foods and dishes, adding to the diversity of your diet.

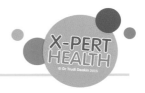

Tip	Why?

5 **Why not try a cheese board for dessert?**

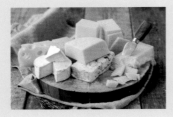

Dairy products are beneficial for our friendly gut bacteria and have been associated with weight loss and a reduced risk of developing a range of diseases such as type 2 diabetes and heart disease.

If you are still hungry after the main meal, why not ask for a cheese board for dessert? You could even share this with others. This will help you keep off high sugar cakes, pastries and desserts and will help you feel fuller for longer. Even better, ask for the cheese to be served on its own or with celery rather than carb-laden items such as crackers, bread or grapes.

6 **If you know you're going to be eating a big meal out, compensate for the remainder of the day**

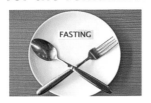

Mix eating out with time-restricted eating (see pages 48 to 51). Having a delicious meal in a restaurant can be very satisfying and it may be easy for you to fast for several hours before the meal so that you can look forward to breaking the fast. Alternatively, you may be so satisfied after the meal that you may be happy to skip breakfast the following morning and not eat again until lunchtime or perhaps the evening meal the next day.

7 **Choose your restaurant wisely!**

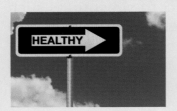

As much as possible, try and choose restaurants where the meal is prepared and cooked using fresh ingredients and is cooked to order.

Try to avoid fast food and large franchised restaurants as these tend to use more processed and refined ingredients. Food is frequently prepared and cooked in bulk and rewarmed on demand in these types of restaurant.

8 **Don't be afraid to request that your food is cooked in butter or olive oil as opposed to vegetable oil**

Ask what fats are used to cook the food. If vegetable oils are used ask if natural fats such as butter, ghee, lard or extra virgin olive oil can be used instead. Many restaurants will accommodate customer wishes and will be happy to do this.

Top 10 Dining Out Tips

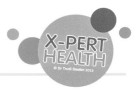

Tip	Why?

9 **Eat slowly and savour your meal**

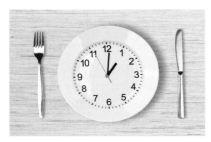

People in Mediterranean countries such as France come together to eat in a relaxed environment over an extended period of time. It tends to be a very sociable event that can reduce stress. The style of eating can therefore be as important for health as what we are eating!

Savour every mouthful and take your time by engaging in conversation. This will allow time for the meal to fill you and will make you less likely to reach for the dessert menu!

10 **Avoid appetisers (bread, breadsticks, crisps etc.)**

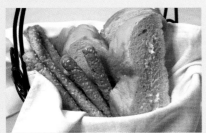

Many appetisers tend to be laden with carbs, which increase insulin levels and drive hunger.

If you are wanting an appetiser why don't you try olives, dips with crudités, antipasti, nuts or even mini tapas to share in place of the usual bread, breadsticks or crisps.

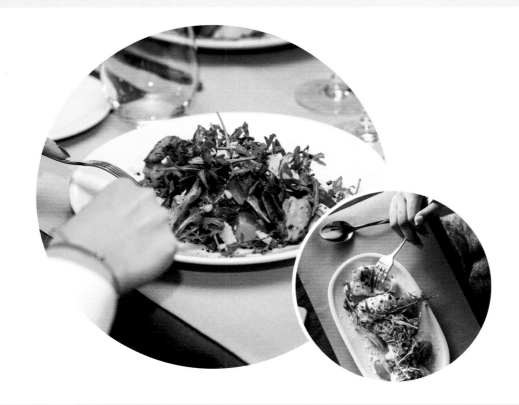

Coping With Bad Days

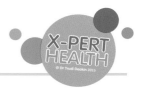

Things don't always go to plan. Dealing with minor set-backs is essential to success. Here are some top tips to help you on your way.

Problem: I ate something believing that it didn't contain carbs but then found out it did

Suggestion: Become more carb aware by looking on food packaging or checking on carb counting lists

Problem: I gave in to my cravings for some carb-containing food

Suggestion: Increase enjoyment of your new dietary approach; for example by trying out new low carb recipes, increasing variety (as sticking to safe foods can be boring) and ensuring that you're having sufficient fat and protein so you aren't left hungry

Problem: I attended a celebration/event and wanted carb-rich foods

Suggestion: There will always be temptations! A small dessert may contain 30-50g of carbs whereas a large portion can contain 50 to 100g. Adopting an 80/20 approach may work for you. This means following your new approach 80% of the time and allowing "slight" slippage to enjoy celebrations without falling off the wagon. However, if you do this too often you will **NOT** see results

Problem: I went out for a meal and there were no reduced carb options on the menu

Suggestion: Accept that you have overconsumed carbs but make sure that you adhere to carb restriction for the rest of the week. Next time ask to replace the carbs (e.g. potato, chips, rice, pasta, bread, chapatti or naan) with vegetables or salad

Problem: I had a chaotic day and just had to grab food on the run

Suggestion: Organisation is the key to success. Plan ahead and pack a breakfast, lunch or evening meal box and take your food with you. Alternately, pop into a convenience store to purchase cheese or cooked meat, fish or seafood to eat with some cherry tomatoes, cucumber or celery sticks. If all else fails you can always practice intermittent fasting!

Problem: I went on holiday and didn't want to think about reducing carbs

Suggestion: Adopting a new dietary approach isn't like being on a diet that you are either on or off – it is a lifelong approach. Although we often wish to leave the day-to-day routine behind, reverting to previous dietary habits will undo all the good you've achieved. **Tailor your dietary approach to your own preferences to maximise your enjoyment of it, and remind yourself on a daily basis what your health goals are and why you want to achieve them!**

Problem: I am an emotional eater and use carbs for comfort depending on my mood (happy, sad, depressed, stressed, upset, excited etc.)

Suggestion: Accepting that you are an emotional eater is a good start. Keep a diary to identify your triggers, i.e. what emotions lead you to overeat, and consider what non-food strategies you can implement to replace food as a response. You cannot change eating behaviour unless you know what is causing it. Try to regain control gradually by setting yourself small and realistic goals. The following pages will discuss how you can identify when you are eating for reasons other than hunger and provides additional tips for you to gain control of this.

Causes Of Hunger

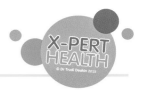

As well as understanding what we should or shouldn't be eating, it is important to understand why we eat. The next few pages consider some of the psychological factors that can affect this, and what we can do to minimise episodes of eating when we aren't truly hungry.

Hunger can come in two main forms:

Physical hunger is the biological urge to eat, driven by certain hormones which stimulate hunger or fullness.

Psychological hunger can be driven by a number of different things, but is usually emotionally based. Paying more attention to the present moment, i.e. to your own thoughts and feelings, can help you to control psychological hunger. Some people call this "mindfulness". Mindfulness can help us enjoy life more and understand ourselves better. If psychological eating is a problem, you can take steps to control it. First you will need to explore the reasons why you are eating when you are not physically hungry.

Possible psychological reasons why we eat:

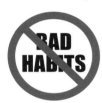

Routine or habit – it is very easy to get into a set eating routine, such as having three meals plus snacks every day. Once a routine has become established it is difficult to break without feeling hungry. Initially, if a meal or snack is omitted, this can lead to psychological hunger and cravings leading to poor food choices.

Boredom – for many people, eating seems like a good solution when there's nothing better to do; whether you graze at home or work, or entertain yourself with lavish dinners out.

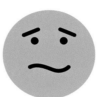

Emotions – eating can be a coping strategy for sadness, loneliness, anger or stress, whereby people often resort to comfort foods. It can also be triggered by happy emotions such as joy and celebrations.

Addiction – some individuals feel "addicted" to food, with similarities to how some people are addicted to certain drugs (see page 65 for more on food addiction). Processed foods, for example, have a powerful effect on the reward centres of the brain.

If you are driven by psychological urges to eat it is highly likely you will be eating carbs to excess, as many popular comfort and snack foods are laden with them. These foods, which tend to be a mix of refined carbs and processed fat, are very easily digested, aren't very filling, and are hyper-palatable (i.e. they are designed to make us want to eat more of them). This leads to overconsumption, high insulin levels and insulin resistance; ultimately causing fat storage and weight gain.

Practicing mindfulness can help you identify what is driving these cravings. Online resources are available from organisations such as Mind UK (https://mind.org.uk/information-support/tips-for-everyday-living/food-and-mood) and the NHS (www.nhs.uk/conditions/stress-anxiety-depression/pages/mindfulness.aspx). Taking control of psychological eating will help you to reduce food intake and improve your health.

Psychology Of Eating

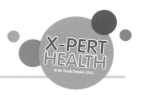

 How do you know if you are eating for psychological reasons?

Some of the tell-tale signs are listed below, but this list is not exhaustive. You may identify additional behaviours that inform you that you are not eating for true hunger:

1. You crave certain foods despite feeling physically full
2. You are constantly preoccupied with food and think about food most of the time
3. When you eat certain foods, e.g. comfort foods, you almost always eat them in large quantities in a short period of time
4. You often eat to the point of feeling uncomfortable and bloated
5. Eating makes you feel out of control and guilty
6. You make excuses (to yourself and others) to justify eating
7. You may hide your eating behaviour from your family, friends and work colleagues
8. You feel more determined to eat healthier foods and lose weight after an uncontrolled eating episode
9. You understand that your eating behaviour is causing health problems but you do not feel like you can control it
10. You can't stop eating at very specific times of the day, e.g. during the evening
11. You often use certain foods as rewards for yourself

If you can relate to several of the reasons listed above, you may have an unhealthy relationship with food and may wish to seek advice from your healthcare team and potentially a psychologist or counsellor. Cognitive behaviour therapy is a talking therapy that can help you manage your problems by changing the way you think and behave. You can see what psychological services are available near you at:

www.nhs.uk/Service-Search/Psychological-therapy-(NHS-IAPT)/LocationSearch/10008

 Tops tips to take charge of psychological eating:

1. Be mindful of what foods you buy. If you do not buy trigger foods then you will not consume them. Try to obtain support from family members to help you remove comfort and snack foods from the house – it'll be better for their health too! If you do buy them for other members of the family, act mindfully by removing them from view and separate into small portions to avoid excessive consumption
2. If you know boredom is a trigger, have a list of strategies in place to keep yourself busy and entertained when you don't have anything else to do. Try to find healthy activities, such as participating in physical activity, to distract yourself when this occurs, as this releases 'feel good' hormones from the brain
3. When you feel hungry consider if the feeling is true hunger or not. Thirst can often be mistaken for hunger. Therefore have a drink to see if the hunger disappears
4. If you start craving food: stop, think and consider what the reasons may be. Adopting a very low carb lifestyle with high quality foods will supply your body with nutrient dense foods that do not spike insulin levels. This will help reduce food cravings
5. Take action to reduce stress and prevent it from becoming a long-term strain impairing your quality of life (see page 66)
6. Ensure you have sufficient good quality sleep (see page 67)
7. Keep a diet diary, noting your mood when you eat. This may help you identify triggers and inform you how different moods affect what and when you eat
8. Do not use food as a reward. Find other ways to do this such as meeting up with a friend, watching a favourite movie or putting the money you would have spent on food into a kitty to save for something special

Carb Addiction

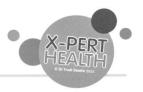

True hunger is controlled by hormones which regulate consumption of essential nutrients; including fats, proteins, vitamins and minerals. This tightly controlled pathway makes foods rich in these nutrients hard to overconsume as they increase levels of fullness hormones. Carbs that are not rich in essential nutrients however activate a different pathway – the endorphin "reward" centre.

The endorphin centre

- Deals with all emotions
- Not regulated by hunger/fullness hormones
- Substances that activate the endorphin pathway need to be consciously controlled
- Endorphins can override the hunger hormones
- No essential nutrient activates the endorphin centre
- Processed carbs and regular snacks activate the endorphin centre, making them very easy to overconsume

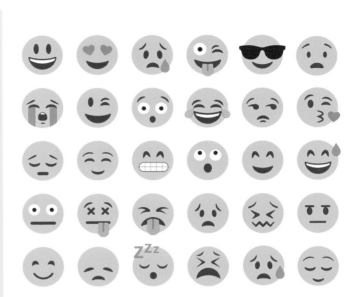

Eating for emotional reasons

Carbs

Foods that activate the endorphin centre can stimulate emotions. This means these foods are often used to deal with emotional stress or as a reward. This can lead to carbs being used when something goes right or wrong in life. Over time this can cause a habit to form.

Eating frequency

Those who eat frequently may be responding to their endorphin "needs" rather than nutritional requirements. Humans typically only need to eat one to three times each day; any more feeds the emotions, not the body. Eating for emotions may lead to addiction-like behaviours over time.

How to reduce or prevent eating for emotional needs:

- Do not use food as a comforter or a reward. Identify other non-food rewards to use instead
- If you do consume carbs only do so as part of a nutritionally dense meal
- Cut out all snacking and do not eat more than three times each day
- Try intermittent fasting (see pages 48 to 51)
- Let true hunger drive your eating behaviour
- Ensure your diet is providing you with all the nutrients you need to prevent cravings

Stress

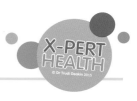

Even if what we are eating is healthy there are a number of non-dietary factors that can have an important influence on our health. The role of stress and sleep are discussed on the next few pages.

What is stress?

Stress is our natural reaction to situations or events that put us under pressure. The feelings we get when high demands are placed on us that are difficult to cope with often lead to stress. Although stress is a normal part of life, if unmanaged high stress levels can lead to an array of problems.

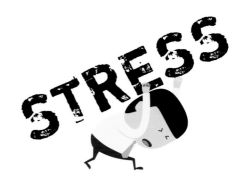

How would we know if we were stressed?

Common signs of stress include feeling:

- Irritable, aggressive or impatient
- Over-burdened
- Anxious, nervous or afraid
- That your thoughts are racing and you can't switch off
- Neglected or lonely
- Depressed
- Disinterested
- That you've lost your sense of humour
- A sense of dread
- Worried about your health
- Unable to enjoy yourself

Physical symptoms can include:

- Shallow breathing or hyperventilating
- Panic attacks
- Blurred eyesight or sore eyes
- Problems getting to sleep or staying asleep; or having nightmares
- Sexual problems, such as losing interest in sex or being unable to enjoy sex
- Feeling tired all the time
- Grinding your teeth or clenching your jaw
- Headaches
- Chest pains
- High blood pressure
- Indigestion or heartburn
- Constipation or diarrhoea
- Feeling sick, dizzy or fainting

What can you do to reduce stress?

Different strategies will work for different people, so it is important to identify a solution that will work for you. Some proven ways to reduce stress are:

- Exercise
- Meditation
- Massage
- Yoga
- Socialising
- Good sleep
- Breathing exercises, for example inhale through your nose for a count of 5, and exhale out of your mouth (as if you're sighing with relief) for a count of 7 or longer. Repeat for at least 90 seconds

If you are struggling to manage stress speak to a healthcare professional, who will be able to signpost you to services that are there to help.

More information about managing stress can be found at:

www.mind.org.uk/information-support/tips-for-everyday-living/stress

www.nhs.uk/Conditions/stress-anxiety-depression/Pages/free-therapy-or-counselling.aspx

Sleep

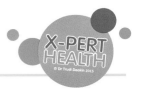

Why is it important to get enough sleep?

Whilst we are asleep our body can perform many essential functions, such as rebuilding muscle tissues that have been worn down during the day and removing toxic byproducts from the body. Sleep can improve our mood, as reward chemicals such as dopamine are released, whilst it can also help create memories because it allows our mind to reflect on the day. Overall, both sleep quality and quantity are vital for restoring our body and mind's ability to function properly.

Sleep deprivation can cause stress hormone levels to rise, leading to an increase in blood glucose, insulin, blood pressure and inflammation. These things can lead to difficulties in managing weight and possibly to longer-term complications.

Having a lack of sleep is also associated with increased appetite and more snacking, with people often turning to processed junk foods as a result. This can cause further weight gain or make it difficult to lose weight, if that is your goal.

Stress can affect our sleep, and a lack of good quality sleep can increase stress levels. This can become a vicious cycle.

What can we do to try and get more sleep, or to improve the quality of the sleep we are getting?

Some tips to improve your sleep include:

- Sleep in complete darkness
- Sleep in loose fitting clothes
- Have a regular sleeping pattern (aim for seven to nine hours per night)
- Keep a cool bedroom
- Stay hydrated, but avoid drinking excessive amounts in the evening
- Avoid using laptops, tablets and phones or watching television just before bed
- Avoid caffeine and alcohol in the evening
- Avoid prolonged daytime naps
- Exercise regularly, but beware that taking part in exercise too late in the evening may interfere with your ability to fall asleep due to the increased release of adrenaline
- Try to relax before bed, for example by having a relaxing bath or shower
- If you wake during the night do not clock-watch. If you're still awake after around 20 minutes get up and engage in a quiet activity such as reading or listening to music until you feel tired, then return to bed

If you are still struggling to sleep after considering these points it may be worthwhile discussing the matter with a healthcare professional.

More information about sleep, and how to improve yours, can be found at:

www.sleepcouncil.org.uk/sleep-advice/

www.healthline.com/nutrition/10-reasons-why-good-sleep-is-important

www.healthline.com/nutrition/17-tips-to-sleep-better

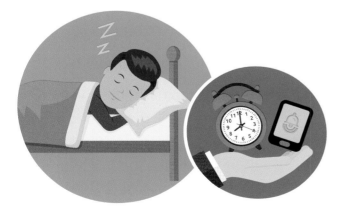

Stress, Sleep And Hormones

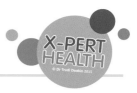

As discussed, high stress levels and poor sleep quality are linked to weight gain. This is in part due to the increase in stress hormones, for example cortisol. Cortisol is released from the adrenal glands when you are stressed and helps to prepare you for 'fight or flight', i.e. to fight the source of stress or run away from it. This provided a huge survival advantage when we were hunter gatherers and came across dangerous animals, but it doesn't offer the same advantages as a response to the types of stress we more commonly experience in today's society.

Stress hormones lead to:

- an increased release of stored glucose from the liver and body cells

- conversion of protein into glucose for energy

Both of these actions lead to raised blood glucose levels, which causes an increase in insulin levels. Elevated insulin levels can increase insulin resistance and fat storage.

Stress hormones are not intended to remain in our blood for long periods of time. Instead, levels should increase and decrease very rapidly. A quick spurt releases instant energy when required (good) but if levels stay raised all day (due to chronic stress or sleep deprivation for example) it results in insulin levels remaining high, causing the body to be in fat storage mode (bad).

What should happen

- Instant energy is required, e.g. to avoid missing a train

- Stress hormone levels increase

- Blood glucose and thus insulin levels increase

- Instant energy becomes available

- You catch the train

- Blood glucose and insulin levels return to baseline

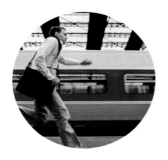

What actually happens

- Everyday stressors, for example at work or at home, become overwhelming

- Stress hormone levels increase

- Blood glucose and thus insulin levels increase

- More immediate energy becomes available

- The stress remains or is replaced with other everyday stressors

- Stress hormone levels remain high

- Insulin levels remain high and insulin resistance develops

- The high insulin levels result in the body being in fat storage mode and weight gain occurs (or weight loss is prevented)

Stress, Sleep And Hormones

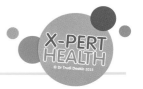

The diagrams on this page outline how the increase in insulin levels caused by elevated stress or a lack of sleep can lead to weight gain. If steps are not taken to tackle stress and/or sleep problems this can become a vicious cycle

Elevated insulin levels mean that fat we eat will be sent to storage, and any fat we already have stored will be kept locked up in our cells. We cannot therefore use any of this energy when insulin levels are high.

This lack of energy availability leads to increased hunger (because the body thinks it needs more fuel) and inactivity (because the body tries to conserve energy). This causes further weight gain, and the continuation of the cycle.

In order to stop this cycle we need to reduce stress levels and/or improve sleep quality and/or quantity. See pages 66 and 67 for a number of strategies that can help.

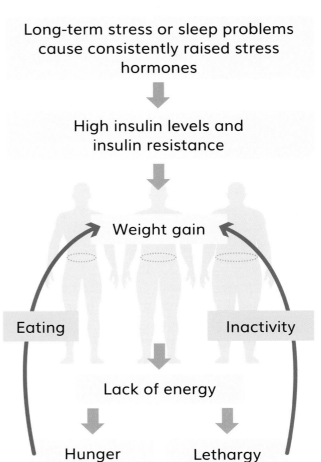

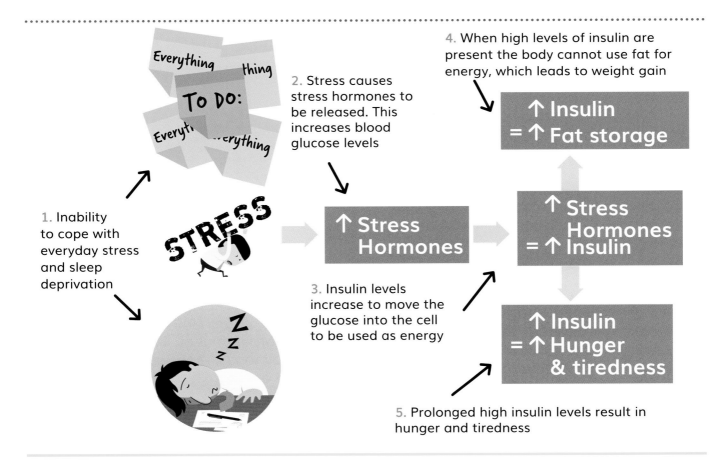

..

Fuelling With Fat

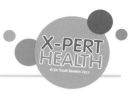

As discussed previously, when restricting carbs it is essential to consume enough fat to make sure you are not hungry all the time. Fat is very misunderstood though, so on the next few pages we discuss different types of fat and why natural, unprocessed fats can be an important part of a healthy dietary approach.

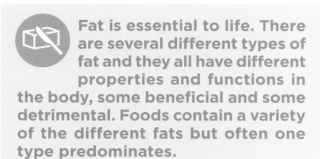

Fat is essential to life. There are several different types of fat and they all have different properties and functions in the body, some beneficial and some detrimental. Foods contain a variety of the different fats but often one type predominates.

Trans fats are found in hydrogenated vegetable oil. Baked goods (especially doughnuts, cookies, cakes and chips) and deep-fried foods are more likely to contain the hydrogenated fat that gives rise to trans fats. Trans fats are harmful, and have been shown to increase heart disease risk. Those most at risk from trans fats are people eating deep-fried takeaway food regularly and/or purchasing cheaper or foreign brands of processed food.

Saturated fat is found in meat, eggs, dairy foods, butter, lard, cheese, cream and coconut oil. Foods that contain large amounts of saturated fat are more likely to be hard at room temperature. Previously thought to cause heart disease, we now know that not all saturated fats have the same effect in our body. There is no need to avoid natural foods that contain some saturated fat. Some natural saturated fats, for example those found in dairy foods, have even been shown to be health promoting.

Dietary cholesterol is found in animal products such as eggs, liver, kidneys and shellfish. Cholesterol is essential in the body. It is a waxy, fat-like substance that performs several important functions: it helps make the outer coating of body cells, it makes up the bile acids that work to digest food in the gut, it has a role in immune function, it allows the body to make

vitamin D, it is needed for the production of hormones, and it is essential for brain function. Consuming dietary cholesterol does not increase blood cholesterol levels in most people, and we now know that it is problems with the transporters that carry cholesterol rather than cholesterol itself that can increase risk of cardiovascular disease (see pages 110 and 111).

Polyunsaturated fat. There are 2 types of polyunsaturated fat. Omega-6 fats are found in seeds and oils like sunflower, safflower, sesame, corn and soya. Omega-3 fats are found in oily fish such as salmon, mackerel and sardines, nuts, cold-pressed rapeseed oil, flaxseeds/linseeds and chia seeds, some pulses, tofu, free-range eggs and grass fed meat. A small amount of both are essential for health, because they cannot be made by the human body. However, the ratio between omega-6 and omega-3 fats is currently too high for most people; largely due to the excessive intake of refined vegetable oils. Too much omega-6 can lead to inflammation, whilst omega-3 has anti-inflammatory properties. Readdressing the balance, by omitting refined vegetable oils and ensuring sufficient intake of omega-3, is beneficial for health.

Monounsaturated fats are widely accepted as healthy. A good source is olive oil (extra virgin is best because heat and chemicals have not been used to extract the oil, see page 74). It is also found in peanut or groundnut oil, whole nuts (such as peanuts, almonds, cashews and Brazil nuts), meat and avocados. Monounsaturated fat protects against cell damage because it is less prone to oxidation and free radical damage than polyunsaturated fatty acids.

Fuelling With Fat

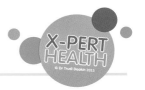

On page 70 we introduced the types of fat we find in the diet, and the main types of foods we might consume that include them. Over the next two pages we will discuss further which of these types of fat should be included as part of a very low carb dietary approach, and which are best avoided. The diagram on page 73 summarises how your diet can influence your CVD risk.

It is recommended that you consume 5-10 portions of fat each day as part of this approach (see page 27). It should be noted however that although this is a high fat diet, some of that fat can come from your own fat stores! When our insulin levels are reduced our body is able to use its stored fat more efficiently for energy, but it wont use this fat if we are consuming too much dietary fat because it will be using the dietary fat instead. If you are struggling to manage your weight despite restricting carbs you may still be consuming too much fat, and so may need to reduce the number of portions you are having.

Red light - avoid

Trans fats are artificial fats that are associated with an increase in heart disease and stroke risk. Consumption of trans fats has gone down significantly in recent years. However, current intake is still high enough to cause harm. In order to avoid trans fats, the best thing you can do is eliminate processed foods from your diet. Some takeaway meals in particular may still contain trans fats.

Processed foods such as chips, crisps, ready meals and biscuits are often a combination of refined carbs and processed vegetable oils. Regular consumption of these foods can cause high blood fat (triglyceride) levels and lead to weight gain. The refined carbs in these foods cause insulin levels to rise, leading to the fat in them being stored in the body. In addition to this, the excess refined carbs are converted to and stored as fat too - making the problem even worse!

Amber light - in moderation

A small amount of omega-6 polyunsaturated fat is essential for life, but there are three reasons why this type of fat should only be eaten in moderation:

1. It is very unstable and prone to damage, resulting in the formation of free radicals. This is bad news in the body as they attack body cells, increasing risk of heart disease and other health problems.

2. Volatile chemicals called aldehydes can be produced when omega-6 polyunsaturated fats are heated, which can further damage the body.

3. It is pro-inflammatory, which means that it encourages long-term inflammation in the body. This damage is the starting point for many diseases.

Therefore the use of refined vegetable oils such as corn and sunflower is discouraged.

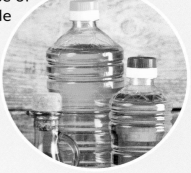

Fuelling With Fat

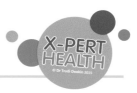

Amber light - in moderation

Saturated fat and dietary cholesterol are not detrimental to health when eaten as part of a real food diet, i.e. when they are a component of natural foods that have not been highly processed. In fact, saturated fat has been shown to increase levels of the HDL particles (road sweepers) that are associated with a reduced risk of CVD (see pages 110 and 111).

No food contains just one type of fat, but real food examples that contain a greater proportion of saturated fat and/or dietary cholesterol include butter, eggs, full fat dairy, shellfish and fatty meats. These foods have not been shown to be detrimental to health, with

growing evidence suggesting that dairy fats in particular may be protective against a number of long-term health conditions.

As far as possible it is preferable to purchase from sources where the animals have been left to roam pastures as this further improves the nutritional profile. Factory farmed animals tend to live in confined spaces, and are often fattened on grain and injected with antibiotics and steroids.

Green light - eat freely (in line with the portion range recommendation for your new dietary approach, see page 27)

Omega-3 polyunsaturated fats are anti-inflammatory, which is the opposite effect to the omega-6 polyunsaturated fats found in vegetable oils. The ratio of omega-6 to omega-3 before the excessive use of vegetable oils was less than 4:1, but this has now risen to around 16:1! Reducing this ratio has been associated with improvements in health outcomes in conditions such as CVD and arthritis. Example of omega-3 containing foods can be found on page 81.

Monounsaturated fat is the predominant fat in both olive oil and rapeseed oil. Research looking at the benefits of olive oil has shown it to lower blood pressure, protect LDL particles from damage, reduce inflammation and help prevent unwanted blood clotting. To obtain the health benefits, olive and rapeseed oils

need to be cold pressed, i.e. extra virgin, as refining using heat and solvents (see page 74) creates the detrimental trans and damaged fats discussed on page 71. In the UK vegetable oil tends to be 100% rapeseed, but this has usually gone through the refinement process and should therefore be avoided.

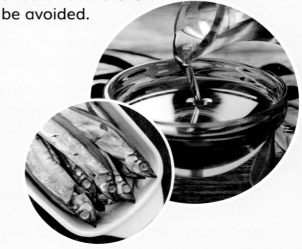

Fuelling With Fat

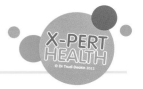

The information from pages 71 and 72, on how fats affect our health, is summarised below.

Foods with processed fats and refined carbs cause blood glucose and insulin levels to rise. This causes fat to be stored in the form of triglycerides (TG) in body cells, including in the liver.

Some of these TG are pushed back out into the blood, leading to the large LDL shrinking to small LDL. Small LDL are more unstable. They are easily damaged, and this results in cholesterol being dropped. This, alongside inflammation (which excess omega 6 can cause), leads to fatty streaks developing in blood vessels.

Over time excess TG leads to the liver becoming fatty and the cells becoming overweight. This causes insulin resistance and further health problems.

Fat containing foods that are not highly processed and are not combined with refined carbs do not cause blood glucose and insulin to rise. They do not therefore lead to an increase in TG levels in the cells or the liver, or a sustained increase in TG levels in the blood.

Saturated fats increase HDL cholesterol, which takes excess cholesterol back to the liver. Omega 3 fats are anti-inflammatory. Monounsaturated fats reduce inflammation and protect LDL particles, preventing them from shrinking and becoming damaged. These types of fat therefore do not increase CVD risk, and may even reduce it.

Legend:
- Small dense LDL-P
- Large bouyant LDL-P
- HDL cholesterol
- Triglycerides
- Glucose
- Insulin

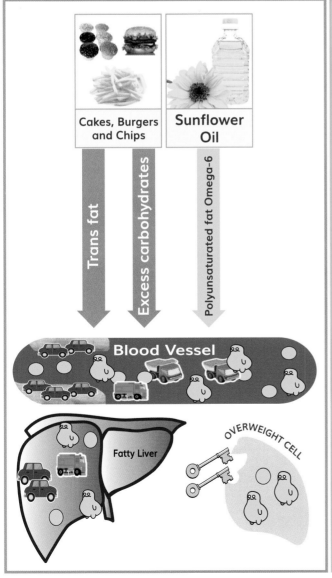

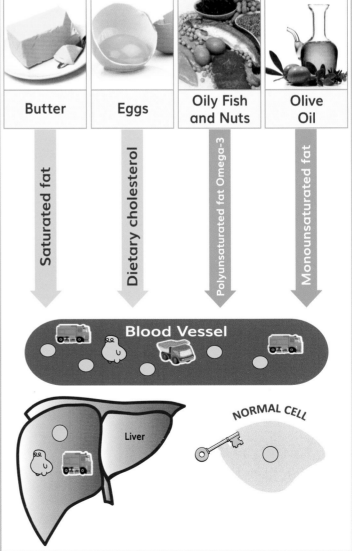

Real Versus Processed Food

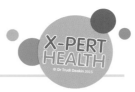

It is advised that processed foods are avoided where possible. Most foods have been processed to a certain extent, although some are clearly more artificially made than others. A summary of some of the key differences between "real" and "processed" foods can be seen in the boxes below:

Real foods:	Processed foods:
• have little or no processing	• have been altered from their natural state
• are as close to their natural state as possible	• have had something taken away from or added to the product
• are nutrient dense	• may have had artificial agents (e.g. preservatives) added and are often packaged in a manner to further extend shelf life, e.g. canned, boxed or bagged
• have had little added or removed for flavouring or preservation	
• are in minimal packaging	• often contain processed fats and sugars or other refined carbs
• have few items on their ingredients list	

Two common examples of products often considered natural and healthy are vegetable oils (processed from seeds) and breakfast cereals (processed from wholegrains). The way they are processed however, which is outlined below, leads to an unnatural product that can be bad for our health.

Vegetable oil:

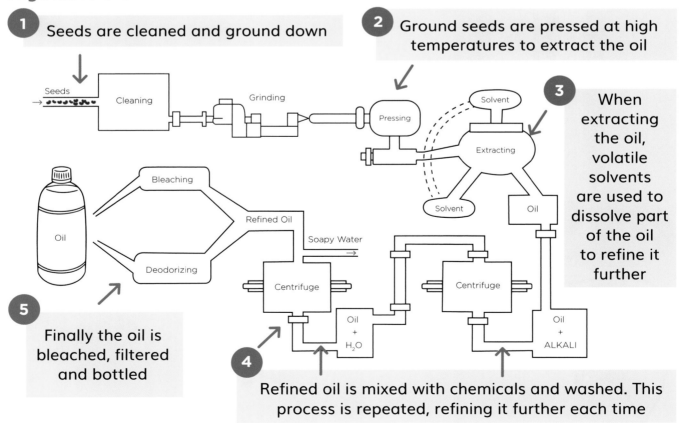

1 Seeds are cleaned and ground down

2 Ground seeds are pressed at high temperatures to extract the oil

3 When extracting the oil, volatile solvents are used to dissolve part of the oil to refine it further

4 Refined oil is mixed with chemicals and washed. This process is repeated, refining it further each time

5 Finally the oil is bleached, filtered and bottled

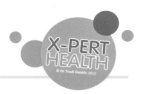

Vegetable oil (continued)

The processing involved in the creation of this product damages the oil and makes it volatile, particularly when heated. The final product is very different to the natural seeds that were used at the start of the process.

Cold pressed and extra virgin monounsaturated oils, e.g. extra virgin olive oil, are much better for you because the oil has been extracted using physical methods and not using heat or solvents.

Breakfast cereals:

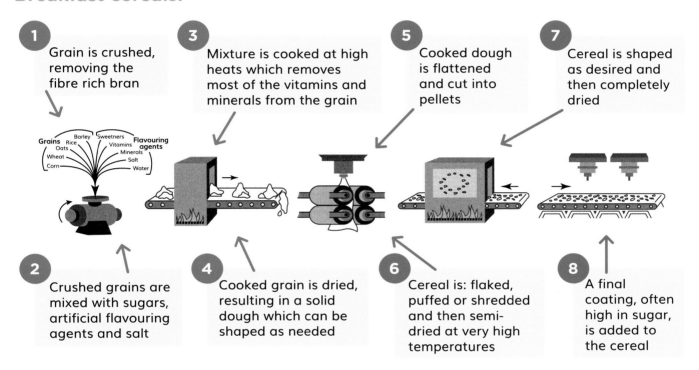

1 Grain is crushed, removing the fibre rich bran

2 Crushed grains are mixed with sugars, artificial flavouring agents and salt

3 Mixture is cooked at high heats which removes most of the vitamins and minerals from the grain

4 Cooked grain is dried, resulting in a solid dough which can be shaped as needed

5 Cooked dough is flattened and cut into pellets

6 Cereal is: flaked, puffed or shredded and then semi-dried at very high temperatures

7 Cereal is shaped as desired and then completely dried

8 A final coating, often high in sugar, is added to the cereal

Grains are small, hard and edible dry seeds that grow on grass-like plants. Today, the most commonly produced and consumed grains are corn (or maize), rice and wheat. A whole grain contains the bran and germ of the grain, which provide fibre and other nutrients. The refining process described above shows how these potentially nutritious parts are removed, leaving only the high-carb section that often gets combined with artificial preservatives, sugar and flavouring agents before being heated at high temperatures and dried. The final product is heavily processed sugary cereals that are digested and absorbed very quickly, leading to rapid spikes in blood glucose and insulin levels causing subsequent hunger and cravings. Some varieties of cereal have had the bran and germ added back in and are therefore classed as wholegrain cereal, but they have still undergone the processing method, to some extent.

It is not recommended to consume breakfast cereal (including wholegrain varieties) when adopting a very low carb dietary approach, as these will make it difficult to keep carb consumption below the 50g target.

Zero And Low Calorie Sweeteners

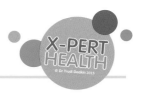

Zero and low calorie sweeteners can replace sugar and therefore reduce your carb intake.

In drinks: You can use the tablets or natural sweeteners as a substitute for sugar in drinks such as tea and coffee.

For baking: Be aware that Stevia or artificial sweeteners are often mixed with bulking agents - typically dextrose or maltodextrin, which are basically glucose!

These products are often much lighter than sugar. To prevent overuse use a tablespoon to measure the sweetener rather than weighing scales when swapping sugar for them. Overuse can cost you a fortune, result in a product that is too sweet, and contain the same amount of carbs as using sugar! **More information about some common sweeteners currently available in the UK is included over the next two pages.**

Natural sweeteners

Natural sweeteners are a good way to reduce carb intake. They do not seem to have any major negative effects, and some may even have a positive impact on your health. They are therefore recommended as an alternative where sweetness is desired. If you have any level of addiction to carbs or sweet flavours however (see page 65) it may be best if you avoid sweeteners altogether, as they can promote cravings for other carb based foods.

Stevia is derived from a plant in South America and has been used for centuries by native Indians in Paraguay. It is a calorie-free herb used as a replacement for sugar and artificial sweeteners. Marketed as a "natural sweetener", manufacturers promote steviol glycosides as a healthier alternative to sugar. It is sold as an herbal powdered extract and is 200-300 times sweeter than sugar.

Acceptable daily intake: 4mg per kg body weight

Brand examples: Stevia, Truvia

Advantages:
• It does not raise blood glucose levels. Although it is absorbed by the body it is rapidly excreted in faeces and urine

• It is extremely heat stable and can be used in cooking and baking

Disadvantages:
• Stevia does not caramelise as sugar does

• The granulated version is often mixed with maltodextrin, which contributes carbs

• Some studies in the 1980's suggested DNA changes occurred when stevia was tested with a certain bacteria. However the European Food Safety Authority (EFSA) has concluded it is safe

• Some people dislike the aftertaste

Sugar alcohols (polyols) including erythritol, mannitol, xylitol and sorbitol are found in some fruits and are also available as sweeteners. Whilst digested slowly, polyols are not fully absorbed into the body and can therefore cause digestive problems in some people if consumed in large amounts or if too much is introduced to the diet too quickly.

Acceptable daily intake: none specified

Advantages:
• About 60 times sweeter than sugar with fewer calories (per gram: sugar 4kcal, erythritol 0.2kcal, mannitol 1.5kcal, xylitol 2.4kcal, sorbitol 2.5kcal)
• Has a clean, cool and pleasant taste
• May be good for dental health
• May be good for your gut microbiota (see page 104)
• Beneficial for people on a reduced carb diet as polyols have very little impact on blood glucose and have been shown to have other beneficial influences on metabolic health

Disadvantages:
• Consuming certain amounts can cause a laxative effect. Like fibre, it may therefore be necessary to introduce it into your diet gradually to build up a tolerance

Zero And Low Calorie Sweeteners

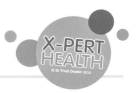

Artificial sweeteners

Artificial sweeteners can help reduce carb intake and so may be a better option than sugar. They are still a processed product however, and so we would not generally recommend their use. There is some evidence that they may not be good for our gut health and may have other negative side effects. However, most of the scare stories related to artificial sweeteners are based on animal studies using very high doses. There is little evidence of any major side effects in humans, but polyols are likely a better option (see page 76).

Aspartame is one of the most popular artificial sweeteners. It is derived from two amino acids (protein building blocks) and is 180-200 times sweeter than sugar.

Acceptable daily intake: 50mg per kg body weight

Brand examples: Canderel, Silver Spoon

Advantages:
• Adds few/no calories to foods and drinks as only a tiny amount needs to be used
• It appears safe for pregnant women

Disadvantages:
• It cannot be used for baking or cooking as it is not stable in heat
• It has been linked to many health concerns; but reviews of the evidence have concluded that it is safe for consumption.

Saccharin is derived from petroleum and is 300-400 times sweeter than sugar. Many foods and drinks (e.g. baked goods, chewing gum and drinks), cosmetic products (e.g. toothpaste), vitamins and medication contain saccharin. It is not broken down when digested. It is slowly absorbed and then rapidly excreted by the kidneys.

Acceptable daily intake: 5mg per kg body weight

Brand examples: Sweetex, Hermesetas

Advantages:
• Adds no calories to foods and drinks
• Can be used in cooking and baking

Disadvantages:
• Some people dislike the aftertaste

Acesulfame-K is a commonly used sweetener that is 200 times sweeter than sugar. It is commonly added to chewing gum, dairy products, drinks and baked goods. It is quickly absorbed, and then excreted through the kidneys, unchanged.

Acceptable daily intake: 9mg per kg body weight

Brand examples: Canderel, Silver Spoon

Advantages:
• It does not affect blood glucose levels
• Adds no calories to foods and drinks
• It can be used in cooking and baking
• It is approved for use during pregnancy

Disadvantages:
• It can leave a bitter aftertaste

Sucralose is 600 times sweeter than sugar. It is usually mixed with maltodextrin, so that it can be used as a substitute for sugar in cooking. It is also found in oral health products (e.g. chewing gum).

Acceptable daily intake: 15mg per kg body weight

Brand examples: Splenda

Advantages:
• Sucralose is calorie-free, and has no effect on blood glucose or tooth decay
• Can be used in cooking and baking

Disadvantages:
• Bulking agents (e.g. maltodextrin) can add around 3g carbs per tablespoon, and this is often not listed on the packaging
• Sucralose can alter the texture of recipes and add an 'artificial' taste

Focus On Alcohol

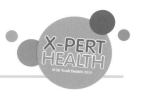

Recommendations: The government advises that people should not regularly drink more than 2-3 units of alcohol a day (equivalent to a pint of 4% beer or a 175ml glass of wine). "Regularly" would mean drinking alcohol every day or most days of the week. The maximum amount of alcohol recommended per week for men and women is 14 units.

The more you drink above the safe limits, the more harmful alcohol is likely to be. Excess consumption can lead to liver disease, pancreatitis, erectile dysfunction, high blood pressure, depression, damage to nerve tissue, some cancers, obesity and addiction.

What is a unit of alcohol? One unit is 10ml or 8g of pure alcohol. It takes the average adult around an hour to process this until there is no alcohol left in their bloodstream, although this varies from person to person.

Alcohol by volume (ABV): Alcohol content is also expressed as a percentage of the whole drink. Look on a bottle of wine or a can of lager and you'll see a percentage, followed either by the abbreviation "ABV", or sometimes just the word "vol". Wine that says "13 ABV" on its label contains 13% pure alcohol.

The alcoholic content in similar types of drinks varies a lot. Some ales are 3.5% but stronger continental lagers can be 5% ABV, or even 6%. The same goes for wine where the ABV of stronger wines can exceed 14%. This means that just one pint of strong lager or a large glass of wine can contain more than three units of alcohol, the upper daily unit guideline limit.

Measures and glass sizes: Spirits used to be commonly served in 25ml measures, which are one unit of alcohol. Many pubs and bars now serve 35ml or 50ml measures. Large wine glasses hold 250ml, which is one third of a bottle. This means there can be three units or more in just one glass. So if you have just two or three drinks, you could easily consume a whole bottle of wine – and almost three times the government's daily alcohol unit guidelines – without even realising. Smaller glasses are usually 175ml and some pubs serve 125ml.

Strategies for drinking less:
- If you drink wine at home, opt for small 125ml glasses and don't fill to the brim.
- Try and pour your own drinks. If your host is constantly topping up your half-filled glass it's hard to keep track of how much alcohol you are drinking.
- Drink spritzers if you like wine, or pints of shandy if you're a lager drinker. You'll still get a large drink, but one that contains less alcohol. To reduce carb load, use sugar-free mixers.
- Opt for half pints if you prefer higher strength lager or try lower strength beer. You may not notice the difference.
- Alternate alcoholic drinks with sugar-free soft drinks.
- If you are uncertain about how much you are drinking, ask the bar staff. Do they pour doubles or singles? How big is their glass of wine?

If you would like to calculate your weekly average, you may find it useful to visit the following website that provides an automated alcohol unit and calorie calculator: **www.drinkaware.co.uk/ understand-your-drinking/unit-calculator** or use the smartphone version of the MyDrinkaware drink tracking tool. It's free and simple to use.

Focus On Alcohol

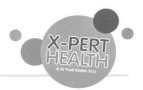

The table below provides alcohol units, calories and carb content for a range of drinks. The carbs are colour-coded green, amber & red for easy reckoning (N.B. As there is large variation between brands, use for general guidance only. Manufacturers also modify the nutritional values from time to time).

Drink	ABV	Units	Calories	Carbs
Red wine - small glass (125ml) e.g. Cote du Rhone, Chianti, Rioja, Shiraz, Merlot & Cabernet Sauvignon	12% to 14.5%	1.5 to 1.8	85-110 kcal	1g
White wine (dry) - small glass (125ml) e.g. Muscadet, Sancerre, Bianco Moncaro, Prosecco	12% to 12.5%	1.5 to 1.6	85-110 kcal	1g
White wine (medium) - small glass (125ml) e.g. Champagnes, Pinot Grigio, Sauvignon Blanc, Chablis, Chardonnay, Cava Brut	11.5% to 13.5%	1.5 to 1.7	85-110 kcal	3g
White wine (sweet) - small glass (125ml) e.g. Sauternes, Moscato	14.5%	1.8	150 kcal	12g
Rose wine - small glass (125ml) e.g. Stowells Light Shiraz, Blossom Hill, Jacob's Creek Shiraz*, Marques De Caceres Rosado	5.5% to 13.5%	0.7 to 1.7	70-126 kcal	1g*- 8g
Fortified wine - pub measure (50ml) e.g. Port, Ruby, Sherry, Special Reserve, Vintage	17.5% to 20%	1	70-80 kcal	3-6g
Whisky - small measure (25ml) e.g. Highland Malt, Scotch, Irish, Bells	40%	1	55 kcal	0g
Brandy - small measure (25ml) e.g. Armagnac, Calvados	40%	1	55 kcal	0g
Gin, Vodka & Rum - small measure (25ml) e.g. Gordons™, Hendrick's™, Greenalls™	37.5% to 40%	1	55 kcal	0g
Cider - 1 pint (568ml) Magners™ Strongbow™	4.5% 5%	2.6 2.8	210 kcal 244 kcal	16g 22g
Alcopops - bottle (275ml) e.g. Smirnoff Ice™ , WKD™	4%	1.1	184 kcal	31g
Lager - 1 pint (568ml) 0% e.g. Becks Blue™, Holsten Alcohol Free™ 4% e.g. Fosters™*,Carling™ Stella Artois™ 5% e.g. Carlsberg Export™, Kronenbourg™*, Peroni™, San Miguel™, Bud bottle™, Grolsch™	0% 4% 5%	0 2.3 2.8	100-140 kcal 170-190 kcal 200-255 kcal	25 - 35g 10*- 15g 12*- 25g
Bitter - 1 pint (568ml) 3.6% e.g. Tetley™ 4% e.g. Boddingtons™*, Wainwrights™	3.6% 4%	2 2.3	187 kcal 170-210 kcal	19g 10*- 20g
Stout e.g. Guinness Draft™	4.1%	2.3	210 kcal	20g

*These are the lower carb alternatives of these drinks

Comparing Foods

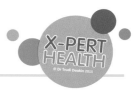

This section compares some of the different varieties of some popular foods, to help you make informed decisions when choosing what to eat.

Chocolate
The darker the chocolate, the lower in carbs and the higher in fibre. Therefore dark bitter chocolate is a better option than milk chocolate. Dark chocolate is also an excellent source of the essential nutrients iron, magnesium, zinc and selenium compared to milk chocolate.

	Milk chocolate 30% cocoa, 100g	Dark chocolate 70% cocoa, 100g	Dark chocolate 99% cocoa, 100g
Calories	622 kcal	566 kcal	590 kcal
Carbs	44g	34g	8g
Sugars	43g	29g	1g
Protein	5g	10g	14g
Fat	47g	41g	51g
Saturated fat	36g	24g	30g
Fibre	0g	12g	20g

Snacks
Although it is best to reduce or omit snacks altogether there are better options than the junk foods many people would usually reach for. Real food options such as nuts are a better option than processed snacks such as biscuits & crisps, because they are much higher in fibre and do not contain refined carbs - though it is important to be mindful of portion sizes as it can still be easy to overconsume nuts.

	Digestive biscuits x2 (30g portion)	Potato crisps per 30g portion	Mixed nuts per 60g portion
Calories	142 kcal	155 kcal	178 kcal
Carbs	19g	17g	6g
Sugars	5g	1g	2g
Protein	1g	1g	10g
Fat	6g	10g	36g
Saturated fat	1.5g	2g	4g
Fibre	0.5g	1g	6g

Comparing Foods

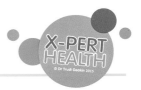

Omega-3

Eating 1 or 2 portions of oil-rich fish per week is advisable as it will provide around 2g to 4g of omega-3 fatty acids. Current average consumption of omega-3 in the UK falls short of the recommended intake. If you don't like oily fish, the table below compares the omega-3 content of a number of other foods and supplements to that of salmon.

Food type	Serving	Omega-3
Oily fish, e.g. salmon	85g	2.6g
Eggs (free range)	2 eggs	0.3g
Milled flax seed	2 tbs	6.7g*
Chia seeds	1 tsp	0.6g*
Cod liver oil extra high strength**	1 capsule	0.4g
	10ml oil	2.3g
Algae oil	1 capsule	0.5g

tbs = tablespoon; tsp = teaspoon

* although non-animal sources can contain omega-3 fatty acids, the body cannot convert them to the beneficial active forms very easily. It may therefore be necessary to consume more of these sources to get sufficient amounts of omega-3

** trials have not shown the consumption of cod liver oil supplements to be effective for reducing CVD risk, so it is probably better to get your omega-3 from real food (although these supplements may still have some benefits, for example they may help reduce pain and stiffness associated with arthritis)

Fats

The table below compares spreads and oils. The processed vegetable oils (sunflower and corn) contain the greater amount of omega-6 fatty acids that are pro-inflammatory and prone to oxidation, which can cause cell damage.

Fat	Butter	Lard	Coconut oil	Olive oil	Rapeseed oil	Sunflower oil	Corn oil
Total	82%	99%	100%	100%	100%	100%	100%
Saturates	52g	40g	87g	14g	7g	12g	14g
Monounsaturates	21g	43g	6g	73g	59g	21g	30g
Polyunsaturates	3g	10g	1.5g	8g	29g	63g	51g
Omega-3 fatty acids	0.7g	0.5g	0g	0.7g	9.6g	0.1g	0.9g
Omega-6 fatty acids	1.4g	9.2g	1.5g	7.5g	19.7g	63g	50g

Starchy Carb Swaps

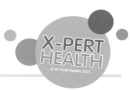

Food - Spaghetti

Low carb version -

Courgette Spaghetti ("Courgetti") or Butternut Squash Noodles ("Boodles")

4 courgettes or 1 butternut squash (600g)

25g butter

10ml extra virgin olive oil

1 clove garlic (crushed)

salt & pepper to taste

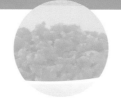

4 servings	8g fat
Per Serving	4g saturates
103 kcal	1.3g salt
3g carbs	
3g fibre	

1. You do not need a spiralizer unless you want even strips
2. Wash, dry, top and tail the courgettes or butternut squash
3. Use a potato peeler to peel strips. Work until you hit seeds and turn the courgette/butternut squash over to do the other side
4. Cut into strips as evenly as you can manage, to your preferred thickness
5. Heat the butter, olive oil and garlic gently. Add courgette/butternut squash and toss around for 4 minutes. Add some freshly ground pepper and a pinch of salt

---

Food - Mashed Potato

Low carb version -

Swede Mash

600g swede

100g butter (or to taste)

salt to taste (1 tsp)

ground nutmeg to taste (optional)

ground black pepper to taste (optional)

you may wish to replace the swede with celeriac

4 servings	
Per Serving	
231 kcal	
8g carbs	
4g fibre	
21g fat	
13g saturates	
1.7g salt	

1. Cut the swede into chunks
2. Put the swede in a large saucepan of salted water. Bring to the boil, then cover and simmer for 20 minutes, until soft
3. Drain in a colander, over a bowl. Keep the water and place the vegetables in a warm serving bowl). Pour a little of the water into the bowl, add the butter and start to mash (optional: if you use a food processor or hand blender, the mash will be smoother)
4. Once mashed, add the nutmeg, salt and black pepper and stir in gently

---

Food - Mashed Potato

Low carb version -

Cauliflower Mash

600g cauliflower, trimmed

100g butter (or to taste)

sea salt to taste (1 tsp)

30g grated parmesan cheese (optional)

60g cream cheese (optional)

4 servings	
Per Serving	
247 kcal	
11g carbs	
3g fibre	
21g fat	
13g saturates	
1.7g salt	

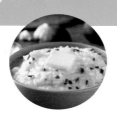

1. Chop the cauliflower, including the core, and add to a large pan of salted boiling water. Cook until completely softened (20-30 minutes)
2. Drain the cauliflower in a colander and press down to remove all the water
3. Transfer the cauliflower to a food processor. Add the butter and puree until completely smooth
4. Return to the pan. Reheat when ready to serve, adding cheese (optional) and salt to taste

Starchy Carb Swaps

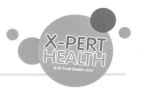

Food - Rice
Low carb version -
Cauliflower Rice

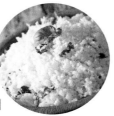

600g cauliflower
salt and pepper
to taste
1 tbs (15ml) olive oil

4 servings
Per Serving
95 kcal
11g carbs
3g fibre
4g fat
1g saturates
1.2g salt

1. Chop cauliflower into small chunks
2. Blend using a food processor or grate the cauliflower until it resembles rice
3. Add to a vegetable stir fry or lightly fry in olive oil for 3-4 minutes

---

Food - Potato crisps
Low carb version -
Kale crisps

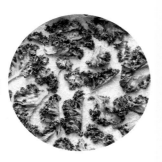

200g kale (thick stems removed)
2 tsp (10ml) olive oil
salt to taste
parmesan to taste (optional)

4 servings   3g fat
Per Serving   1g saturates
43 kcal   0.5g salt
1g carb
2g fibre

1. Preheat the oven to 140°C/120 °C fan/ gas 1
2. Tear the kale into pieces and toss together with olive oil to coat
3. Spread the kale out over 2 baking trays, making sure the leaves don't touch
4. Scatter with salt (this step can be done now, or after removing from the oven)
5. Cook for 10 minutes, then turn and cook for a further 15 minutes until crisp
6. Sprinkle with parmesan (optional)
7. Remove from the oven and store in an airtight container for up to 3 days

---

Food - Roast Potatoes
Low carb version -
Roast Vegetables

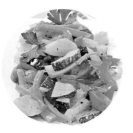

300g swede
300g courgette
2 peppers
1 tbs (45g) goose fat
salt to taste

4 servings   5g fibre
Per Serving   12g fat
165 kcal   3g saturates
9g carbs   1.2g salt

1. Pre-heat the oven to 200°C/180°C fan/ gas 6
2. Peel and chop the swede and add to a large pan of water. Cook until the edges are slightly soft (5-10 minutes)
3. Drain in a colander and toss to make edges fluffy
4. Slice courgettes and peppers and combine with the other vegetables
5. Pour all vegetables into an oven tray and add the goose fat
6. Mix to ensure goose fat covers all the vegetables and cook for 50 minutes (occasionally stirring throughout)

Starchy Carb Swaps

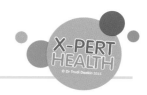

Food - Chips

Low carb version - Spicy Carrot Fries

600g fresh carrot

1 tbs ground black pepper

1 tbs cayenne pepper

lard (for deep frying)

salt to taste (1 tsp)

4 servings	13g fat
Per Serving	5g saturates
178 kcal	1.3g salt
12g carbs	
6g fibre	

Carb content can be further reduced by using either swede or celeriac instead of carrots

1. Turn on a deep fat fryer to melt lard
2. Peel and slice carrots
3. Boil sliced carrots in salt water to soften (10-15 minutes)
4. Drain in a colander and add to the deep fat fryer
5. Fry carrots until outsides are crispy (10-12 minutes)
6. Drain fries of excess lard and tip into a warm bowl
7. Mix in salt, black pepper and cayenne pepper to taste

Food - Mac 'n' Cheese

Low carb version - Cauliflower Cheese

80g grated cheddar

300ml double cream

100ml water

600g cauliflower

30g grated parmesan (or more cheddar)

salt to taste

pepper to taste

4 servings	50g fat
Per Serving	31g saturates
547 kcal	1g salt
12g carbs	
3g fibre	

1. Gently simmer double cream and water (mixed) for 5-8 minutes, adding salt and pepper to taste
2. Remove from the heat, stir in the cheddar and allow to melt
3. Set sauce aside and chop cauliflower into separate small heads
4. Pre-heat the oven to 200°C/180°C fan/gas 6
5. Place cauliflower into an oven dish and top with cheese sauce
6. Bake for approximately 30 minutes until the cauliflower is soft, then sprinkle cheese over the top and return to the oven for a further 10-15 minutes
7. Serve, adding salt and pepper to taste

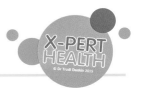

Food - Pancakes

Low carb version -
Fluffy Almond Flour Pancakes

2 eggs (separated)
175g almond flour
1 tsp baking powder

125ml double cream
125ml water
butter (to fry in)

10 servings
Per Serving
201 kcal
2g carbs
2g fibre
19g fat
6g saturates
0.3g salt

1. Separate the egg yolks from the whites
2. Whisk the whites until they form stiff peaks
3. Whisk the almond flour, baking powder, egg yolks, cream and water to form a thick batter
4. Fold in the peaked egg whites
5. Cover the mixture with cling film and place in a fridge for one hour
6. After the mixture has been allowed to rest, melt the butter in a large pan and ladle the batter into the pan to form small 10cm pancakes
7. Fry until bottoms are golden brown (3-4 minutes) then flip the pancakes and cook for a further 2 minutes
8. Serve with your favourite ingredients (e.g. Greek yoghurt and mixed berries)

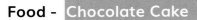

Food - Chocolate Cake

Low carb version - Low Carb Chocolate Cake

Cake:

200g erythritol
200g butter
4 eggs
175g ground almonds
2 tsp baking powder
25g cocoa powder

Icing:

300ml double cream (whipped)
50g dark chocolate (70% to 99% cocoa solids)

12 servings
Per Serving
397 kcal
2g carbs
2g fibre
40g fat
20g saturates
0.4g salt

1. Pre-heat the oven to 180°C
2. Grease a suitable cake tin or alternatively cover the inside with baking parchment
3. Beat the erythritol and butter together to form a creamy paste
4. Continue beating, adding the eggs one at a time
5. Fold in the ground almonds, baking powder and cocoa powder
6. Pour the mixture into the cake tin and bake for 25-35 minutes, until the top of the cake is slightly brown. A skewer should come out clean
7. Leave to cool in the tin
8. Whip the double cream until soft peaks are formed
9. Either cover or fill the centre of the cake with the whipped cream and grate the chocolate as desired

(alternatively melt the dark chocolate and combine with the whipped cream prior to spreading over the cake, adding a small amount of erythritol – if desired)

For more recipes check out the free X-PERT Health online forum, at www.xperthealth.org.uk/forums

Low Carb Recipes

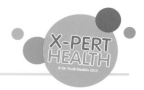

English Muffin (2 minutes microwave)

1 egg

1 tbs water

1 tbs olive or coconut oil

3/4 tsp baking powder

1 heaped tbs (30g) ground almonds

1 heaped tbs (20g) golden flax seed (milled)

1 pinch sea salt

optional: 1 tsp of seeds such as chia seeds

Serving suggestion: slice horizontally and toast or fill with your favourite ingredients

1. In a small glass dish or ramekin, whisk egg with the oil and water
2. Whisk in remaining ingredients
3. Microwave on high for two minutes or until the muffin feels firm to the touch
4. Leave to cool

1 serving:	10g fibre
Per Serving	44g fat
499 kcal	5g saturates
3g carbs	1.6g salt

Low carb thin & crispy pizza

200g mozzarella cheese, shredded

100g cheddar cheese, grated

3 eggs

1 tsp garlic powder

1 tsp dried basil, optional

Toppings: 75g pepperoni, 75g salami, 100g mushrooms, 100g green peppers, 200g passata, 100g mozzarella cheese

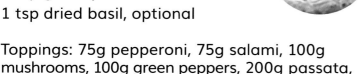

1. Mix the cheeses, eggs, garlic powder and basil well
2. Either grease a 16-inch pizza pan or line with greaseproof paper/ nonstick foil
3. Evenly spread the cheese mixture in the pan, almost to the edge, making it as thin as possible
4. Bake at 200°C for 15-20 minutes until golden brown
5. Spread passata, toppings and cheese. Keeping the oven rack in the center position, put the pizza under the grill until the cheese is melted and bubbly, about 4-5 minutes

4 servings	2g fibre
Per 271g Serving	43g fat
591 kcal	20g saturates
8g carbs	3g salt

Serving suggestion: Add variety by adding different toppings each time you make it.

Ground Almond & Walnut Scones

250g ground almonds

2 tsp baking powder

100g walnut pieces (alternatively you can use pecans)

50g butter

1 egg (beaten)

2 tbs sweetener

pinch of salt

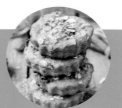

10 (52g) servings:
Per Serving
269 kcal
2g carbs
4g fibre
26g fat
4g saturates
0.7g salt

1. Mix the dry ingredients
2. Melt the butter and add to dry ingredients
3. Add sufficient beaten egg until a dough is formed
4. Portion into 10 scones
5. Place on a baking tray and cook in a moderately hot oven (180°C) for approximately 20 minutes until set and golden brown

The recipe can be adapted by adding a small amount of cocoa powder to make chocolate scones or adding 25g psyllium husk powder to increase the fibre content

Low Carb Recipes

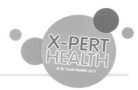

Almond & parmesan chicken/fish goujons

1 or 2 eggs
500g raw chicken/fish fillets (cut into strips)
50g grated parmesan cheese
50g ground almonds
Salt & pepper to taste, spices optional
Lard for frying

4 (192g) servings:	2g fibre
Per Serving	27g fat
416 kcal	9g saturates
1g carbs	1g salt

1. Whisk eggs together in a bowl
2. Dunk chicken/fish strips in the egg. Shake off any excess
3. Mix parmesan and ground almonds in another bowl. Add spices
4. Roll the strips in this coating mixture. Set on a plate for 10 minutes
5. Melt lard in a deep frying pan or deep fat fryer. Fry strips for 8-15 minutes until cooked through, golden brown and crispy

N.B. The coating mixture can be used to coat other foods such as prawns or mushrooms.

Aubergine and cashew bake

2 aubergines (500g)
6 tbsp (100ml) olive oil
100g raw unsalted cashews
50g fresh coriander
2 cloves of garlic, minced

4 servings	4g Fibre
Per Serving	38g Fat
402kcal	6g saturates
7g carbs	0.1g Salt

Serving suggestion: Vary the toppings!

1. Preheat the oven to 170°C
2. Slice aubergines in half and place, sliced side up, on a baking tray. Drizzle with oil.
3. Bake until tender (approx. 25 minutes)
4. Blend cashews, coriander, garlic and 6 tbsp of olive oil to form a chunky paste. Add water if necessary.
5. Spread the paste on top of the aubergines. Grill until golden.

Chicken, cream cheese and bacon

4 boneless chicken fillets (520g)
150g garlic & herb full fat soft cheese
20g butter
4 slices of streaky bacon
Salt & pepper to taste

4 servings:	0g fibre
Per Serving	19g fat
325 kcal	11g saturates
1g carbs	2.1g salt

1. Preheat the oven to 200°C
2. Cut an insert into each chicken breast
3. Spread cream cheese inside each chicken breast and dot with butter
4. Wrap a bacon slice around each chicken fillet and secure with a toothpick
5. Bake for 35-40 minutes until juices run clear and bacon is crispy

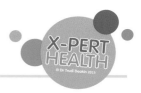

Spinach* frittata

9 large eggs

2 tbsp (30ml) double cream

2 tbsp (34g) sun-dried tomatoes, chopped

Salt and freshly ground pepper to taste

1 medium onion (150g), chopped

1 large clove garlic, minced

2 tbsp (30ml) extra-virgin olive oil

500g spinach leaves, chopped

80g goats cheese

4 (336g) servings:	7g fibre
Per Serving	34g fat
440 kcal	11g saturates
6g carbs	1.7g salt

1. Preheat oven to 200°C. Whisk eggs and cream together in a bowl, add sun-dried tomatoes, salt and pepper
2. Sauté onions and garlic in olive oil in an oven-proof, non-stick frying pan, until translucent. Add the spinach and cook for 2-3 minutes
3. Spread out this mixture evenly and cover with egg mixture. Lift up the spinach with a spatula to let the egg flow underneath
4. Sprinkle with goats cheese. When the frittata is half set, put the pan in the oven. Bake for 13-15 minutes until puffy and golden

* Frittata can be made with a variety of options by swapping the spinach with, for example, smoked salmon, tuna, onions, pepper or blue cheese

Beef lasagne with leek pasta

2 large (600g) leeks

50g butter

1 onion, chopped

2 garlic cloves, crushed

500g minced beef

3 peppers, chopped

150g mushrooms, chopped

150ml red wine

200ml beef stock, using 1 beef stock cube

200g can chopped tomatoes

2 tbsp (100g) tomato purée

2 tubs (400g) full fat soft cheese

50g extra-mature cheddar, grated

25g parmesan, finely grated

1 tsp dried oregano, 2 bay leaves, salt & pepper

6 servings:	42g fat
Per 478g Serving	24g saturates
582 kcal	1.6g salt
15g carbs	
6g fibre	

1. Trim leeks to the width of the lasagne dish. Cut length ways, open them out and separate out the larger outer leaves- these will be your 'lasagne' sheets
2. Fry garlic & onion in butter in a non-stick pan. Add minced beef, peppers and mushrooms. Cook for 5 minutes
3. Add red wine, beef stock, tomatoes, tomato puree, oregano and bay leaves. Bring to a simmer for 30 minutes and season
4. Add 'lasagne' to a half-filled saucepan of boiling water. Bring to the boil and cook for 5 minutes. Drain and dry on kitchen paper when cold
5. Place the mince mixture and leeks in the dish in alternating layers
6. Melt soft cheese in a pan and add cheddar. Bring to a simmer. Cook for 5 minutes until thick and smooth, stirring regularly
7. Pour the sauce over the lasagne and sprinkle with parmesan. Bake for 30 minutes at 200°C

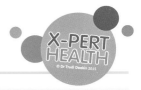

Steak and kidney pie with almond crust

For the crust
200g ground almonds / 50g coconut oil or butter (melted) / pinch of salt / beaten egg

For the filling
50g butter
700g stewing beef, diced
200g lamb kidney, diced
2 medium onions, diced
850ml beef stock
15g golden milled flaxseed
Salt, pepper, 1tbsp Worcestershire sauce

6 servings:	6g fibre
Per 407g Serving	43g fat
595 kcal	14g saturates
8g carbs	1.6g salt

1. Melt coconut oil/butter. Add almonds and salt. Mix to a dough and refrigerate for 30 minutes
2. Heat butter in a pan and brown the beef. Set aside. Brown kidneys in the pan, add onions and cook for 3-4 minutes
3. Re-add the beef. Add stock and flaxseed. Stir until brought to the boil. Simmer for 1 ½ hours
4. Remove from the heat. Add salt, pepper and Worcestershire sauce. Allow to cool completely before placing into a pie dish
5. Roll out the pastry (between 2 sheets of cling film) to the pie dish size and 5mm thick
6. Place pastry over the dish. Trim and crimp edges
7. Brush with beaten egg. Bake for 30-40 minutes at 200°C until golden

Chicken curry

4 chicken breasts (520g), diced

Sliced vegetables (1 onion, 1 red pepper, 1 stalk celery)

1 clove garlic, crushed

1 tsp each ground spices: turmeric, curry powder, ginger

1 tbs milled flaxseed or coconut flour

1 pint chicken stock

60g crème fraîche or double cream

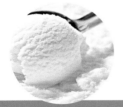

4 servings:	3g fibre
Per 393g Serving	12g fat
275 kcal	6g saturates
6g carbs	2.4g salt

1. Fry chicken until browned, add vegetables and garlic and cook for 10 minutes. Add spices and flaxseed or flour. Cook for 2 minutes
2. Add in the chicken stock and stir thoroughly, simmer for 20-30 minutes
3. Take off the heat. Stir in crème fraîche/cream

Ice cream
4 egg yolks
4 tbsp sweetener*
1tsp vanilla essence**
500ml double cream

6 servings:	0g fibre
Per 106g Serving	48g fat
454 kcal	29g saturates
1g carbs	0.1g salt

1. Beat egg yolks, sweetener and vanilla essence with an electric mixer until pale and creamy
2. Whip cream in another bowl until soft peaks form
3. Gently fold in sweetener/egg yolk mix
4. Pour into plastic container with a tight fitting lid and freeze overnight

* see pages 76 and 77 for more about sweeteners. Where sweeteners are included in recipes natural sweeteners are better options than artificial ones. If using erythritol for this ice cream recipe use a powdered variety to avoid the end product having a grainy feel

** You can swap the vanilla essence for a different flavouring, for example for melted chocolate, coffee, or pureed berries

Low Carb Recipes

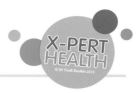

Cheesecake

75g butter (chopped)

250g ground almonds

2 tbs granulated sweetener

3 eggs

3 tbs granulated sweetener

Rind and juice of large lemon

500g cream cheese (full fat)

14g gelatine soaked in 3 tbsp water

100ml double cream

8 servings:	4g fibre
Per 169g Serving	49g fat
515 kcal	21g saturates
4g carbs	0.7g salt

1. Rub butter into almonds & sweetener. Mould into base of cake tin
2. Bake at 200°C for 10-15 minutes
3. Separate eggs. Add sweetener and lemon rind to yolks and beat. Add cream cheese and lemon juice. Beat
4. Soak gelatine in water for 5 minutes and then gently heat until dissolved
5. Add gelatine mix to cream cheese
6. Lightly whip cream until firm. Stir into cream cheese mix. Beat egg whites until stiff. Fold into mix
7. Cover almond base with cream cheese mix. Refrigerate until set

Chocolate Cake (3 minutes microwave)

4 tbs (120g) ground almonds

1 tbs (30g) cocoa

1/2 tsp (2g) baking powder

1 tbs granulated sweetener

2 tbs (60g) melted butter

1 tbs water

1 egg

4 servings:	5g fibre
Per 76g Serving	30g fat
319 kcal	9g saturates
3g carbs	0.5g salt

1. Mix almonds, cocoa, baking powder and sweetener in a bowl
2. Stir in the melted butter, water and egg. Mix well with a spoon or fork
3. Scrape batter down evenly with a spatula. Cover with cling film and vent by cutting a small slit in it
4. Microwave on HIGH for 1 minute to 1 minute 20 seconds until set but still a little moist on top

Chocolate filled ginger biscuits

200g ground almonds

2 tbs granulated sweetener

1 tsp ground ginger & cinnamon

1 tsp baking powder & 1/4 tsp salt

1 large egg, beaten

2 tbs butter, melted & 2 tsp vanilla extract

Chocolate filling: 5 tbs butter / 50g chocolate (80% cocoa) / 2 tbs sweetener / 25g cocoa / 1/4 tsp vanilla extract

15 servings:	2g fibre
Per 45g Serving	21g fat
212 kcal	9g saturates
2g carbs	0.4g salt

1. Whisk together almonds, sweetener, ginger, cinnamon, baking powder and salt. Add egg, butter and vanilla
2. Form a dough and roll out (1/2cm thick). Cut into circles (5cm diameter) and place on baking sheet
3. Bake for 15 minutes at 150°C until firm and golden
4. Melt butter, chocolate and sweetener over a low heat. Add cocoa and vanilla and whisk. Remove from heat
5. When cool, add filling between 2 cookies

Carb Awareness Of Everyday Foods

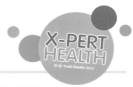

Pages 91 to 100 show the carb content and impact on blood insulin of 165 commonly consumed foods and drinks.

less than 2g per portion (no impact on insulin levels)	2g to 10g per portion (small impact on insulin levels)
11g to 25g per portion (medium impact on insulin levels)	more than 25g per portion (large impact on insulin levels)

Food/drink	Food image		Carb content per 100g	Portion size	Carbs per portion (g)	Impact on insulin levels
Apples (1 small)			11.8	130g	15.3	Medium
Banana (1 small, 80g peeled / 128g with skin)			23.2	80g	18.5	Medium
Blueberries (4 heaped tablespoons)			6.9	80g	5.5	Small
Broccoli (2-3 tablespoons)			1.8	80g	1.4	No impact
Butternut squash (2-3 tablespoons)			7.1	80g	5.7	Small
Celeriac (2-3 tablespoons)			2.3	80g	1.8	No impact
Carrots (2 tablespoons)			6.1	80g	4.9	Small
Dried fruit (raisin or apricot, 1 dessert spoon)			67.2	25g	16.8	Medium
Grapes (approx. 12)			15.4	80g	12.3	Medium
Mango (3-4 slices)			13.8	70g	9.7	Small
Mediterranean roasted vegetables (2-3 tablespoons)			6.2	80g	5	Small
Orange juice (1 medium glass)			8.8	250ml	22	Medium
Peaches in juice, (2 tablespoons)			18	125g	14.5	Medium
Peas (mushy processed, 2 tablespoons)			13.1	100g	13.1	Medium
Peas (frozen, 2-3 tablespoons)			11	80g	9	Small
Soup - vegetable cup (1 sachet)			5.5	218ml	12	Medium

fruit & vegetables

Carb Awareness Of Everyday Foods

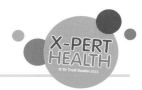

Food/drink	Food image	Carb content per 100g	Portion size	Carbs per portion (g)	Impact on insulin levels
Strawberries (approx. 7)		5.9	80g	4.7	Small
Swede (2-3 tablespoons)		2.3	80g	1.8	No impact
Sweetcorn (2 tablespoons)		16.9	80g	14	Medium
Tomatoes (chopped, ½ can)		4	200g	8	Small
Tomatoes (1 raw)		3.1	80g	2.5	Small
Bulgur wheat (½ cup, uncooked)		20.3	75g	15.2	Medium
Bread - garlic (¼ small baguette)		44	53g	23.3	Medium
Bread - low carb mix (1 slice of bread)		3.6	30g	1.1	No impact
Bread - cinnamon & raisin bagel (1 average)		50.1	90g	45.1	Large
Bread - naan (1)		46	90g	41.4	Large
Bread - pitta (1)		47.9	60g	28.5	Large
Bread - seeded roll (1)		40.9	72g	29.4	Large
Bread - soya & linseed (1 slice)		27.3	33g	9	Small
Bread - tortilla wrap (1)		50.2	62g	31.1	Large
Bread - white (1 slice)		44.5	40g	17.8	Medium
Bread - wholemeal (1 slice)		38.5	40g	15.4	Medium
Breadstick (1)		57.2	8g	4.6	Small
Breakfast biscuits (2)		68	25g	17	Medium

 fruit & vegetables   starchy carbs

www.xperthealth.org.uk

Carb Awareness Of Everyday Foods

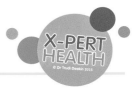

less than 2g per portion (no impact on insulin levels)	2g to 10g per portion (small impact on insulin levels)	11g to 25g per portion (medium impact on insulin levels)	more than 25g per portion (large impact on insulin levels)	

Food/drink	Food image	Carb content per 100g	Portion size	Carbs per portion (g)	Impact on insulin levels
Cereal - brunch bar, raisin (1)		65	32g	21	Medium
Cereal - chocolatey squares (1 small bowl)		64.7	30g	19.4	Medium
Cereal - Cornflakes™ (1 small bowl)		84	30g	25	Medium
Cereal - porridge oats (3-4 tablespoons)		70.8	50g	35.4	Large
Cereal - Shredded Wheat™ bitesize (1 small bowl)		68.7	40g	27.5	Large
Cereal - Swiss style muesli (2 tablespoons)		62.5	45g	28.1	Large
Cereal - wheat bisks (2)		69	37g	25.5	Large
Chapatti (1 small)		46.3	45g	20.8	Medium
Crispbread - mixed grain (2 crackers)		66.7	19g	12.6	Medium
Crumpet (1)		39.5	46g	18.2	Medium
Pasta - spaghetti (½ chilled packet, cooked)		29.7	280g	83.1	Large
Pizza (½ pepperoni deep pan)		31	200g	62	Large
Pizza (½ thin crust cheese feast)		29.7	128g	38	Large
Potato (boiled, 3 egg-sized)		16.1	100g	16.1	Medium
Potato (mashed, ½ pack -200g)		13.7	200g	27.4	Large
Potato (oven chips)		24	134g (cooked)	32	Large

🍞 starchy carbs

Carb Awareness Of Everyday Foods

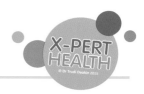

Food/drink	Food image	Carb content per 100g	Portion size	Carbs per portion (g)	Impact on insulin levels
Rice - Chinese style (½ pack)		27.1	140g	37.9	Large
Rice (½ microwave packet)		30.9	125g	38.6	Large
Rice noodles (½ pack)		25.9	188g	48.6	Large
Biscuits - chocolate fingers (4)		60	21g	12.6	Medium
Biscuits - rich tea (2)		71.1	16.6g	11.8	Medium
Biscuits - digestives (2)		62.9	29.6g	18.6	Medium
Biscuits - Twix™ (2 fingers)		64.6	50g	32.2	Large
Bombay mix (small handful)		50	40g	20	Medium
Cake - chocolate (1 very small slice)		53.5	64g	34	Large
Chocolate - coffee creams (2)		76.9	18g	14.2	Medium
Chocolate- Dairy Milk™ (4 chunks)		56.5	22.5g	12.5	Medium
Chocolate - dark 85% cocoa (3-6 squares)		26.4	20g	5.3	Small
Chocolate - no added sugar (6 squares)		49.7 (polyols 33.1)	25g	Available 4.1	Small
Chocolate - fancy filled (2)		64	26g	16.6	Medium
Crisps - Doritos™ (approx ½ 66g pack)		55.4	30g	16.6	Medium
Crisps (1 bag)		52	30g	15.6	Medium
Crisps - hand-cooked (¼ 150g pack)		49	37.5g	18.4	Medium
Dessert - blackcurrant & Madagascan vanilla (1)		39.4	73g	28.7	Large

🈸 starchy carbs   🔲 sugary carbs

www.xperthealth.org.uk

Carb Awareness Of Everyday Foods

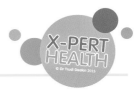

	less than 2g per portion (no impact on insulin levels)		2g to 10g per portion (small impact on insulin levels)		11g to 25g per portion (medium impact on insulin levels)		more than 25g per portion (large impact on insulin levels)

Food/drink	Food image	Carb content per 100g	Portion size	Carbs per portion (g)	Impact on insulin levels
Dessert - coconut milk with pineapple & chilli (1)		21	100g	21	Medium
Dessert - strawberry trifle (¼ pack)		17.4	150g	26.1	Large
Fizzy drink - Coca Cola™ (1 can)		10.6	330ml	35	Large
Fizzy drink - Diet Coca Cola™ (1 can)		0	330ml	0	No impact
Fizzy drink - Lucozade™ (1 bottle)		8.9	380ml	33.8	Large
Fizzy drink - sugar free (1 can)		0.6	500ml	3	Small
Hot chocolate drink (1 sachet)		69.3	25g	17.3	Medium
Ice cream - Magnum Classic™ (1)		29	79g	23	Medium
Ice cream - Magnum White™ (1)		33	79g	26	Large
Ice cream - vanilla (1 scoop)		23.2	55g	12.7	Medium
Jaggery Goor - cane sugar (1 matchbox-size chunk)		95	30g	28.5	Large
Jam - reduced sugar (1 teaspoon)		43	15g	6.5	Small
Jam - strawberry (1 teaspoon)		60.5	15g	9.1	Small
Jelly - sugar-free (1 sachet)		15.6	23g sachet	0.4	No impact
Sweetener - artificial (Splenda, 1 tsp)		97.7	0.5g	0.5	No impact
Sweetener - polyol (xylitol or erythritol, 1 tsp)		100g (polyol)	5g	No available carbs	No impact

sugary carbs

Carb Awareness Of Everyday Foods

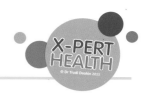

Food/drink	Food image	Carb content per 100g	Portion size	Carbs per portion (g)	Impact on insulin levels
Sweets - Haribo™ (mini pack)		79	40g	31.6	Large
Sweets - Indian - gulabjam (1 sweet)		48.1	83g	40	Large
Sweets - Liquorice Allsorts™ (4 sweets)		77.8	25g	19.5	Medium
Tarts - cherry Bakewell (1 tart)		65.6	48g	31.2	Large
Benecol™ (1 bottle)		7.1	67.5g	4.8	Small
Cheese - light cheese spread (1 portion)		6.5	17.5g	1.2	No impact
Cheese - mature cheddar (matchbox-size chunk)		0.1	30g	0	No impact
Cheese - Philadelphia™ soft cheese (1 dessert spoon)		5.1	30g	1.5	No impact
Cheese - reduced fat cheddar (matchbox-size chunk)		3	25g	0.8	No impact
Cheese - blue (small matchbox-size)		0.4	30g	0.1	No impact
Custard - instant - just add water (1/3 packet made up)		16.8	26g powder	19	Medium
Milk (1/3 pint)		4.8	200ml	9.6	Small
Yoghurt - fruit bio live organic (1 pot)		13.6	150g	20.4	Medium
Yoghurt - Greek fruit (1 pot)		15.7	110g	17.3	Medium
Yoghurt - Greek natural full fat (3 tablespoons)		4.9	150ml	7.4	Small
Yoghurt - Muller Light™ strawberry fat free (1 pot)		7.8	175g	13.7	Medium
Butter (2 level teaspoons)		0.8	10g	0	No impact
Coconut oil (3 level teaspoons)		0	10g	0	No impact

 sugary carbs   Dairy   fats

www.xperthealth.org.uk

Carb Awareness Of Everyday Foods

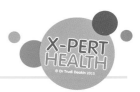
X-PERT HEALTH
© Dr Trudi Deakin 2015

	less than 2g per portion (no impact on insulin levels)		2g to 10g per portion (small impact on insulin levels)		11g to 25g per portion (medium impact on insulin levels)		more than 25g per portion (large impact on insulin levels)

Food/drink	Food image	Carb content per 100g	Portion size	Carbs per portion (g)	Impact on insulin levels
Cream - double (2 tablespoons)		1.6	30ml	0.5	No impact
Dips - various		5.6	133g	7.5	Small
Goose fat (2 teaspoons)		0	10g	0	No impact
Lard (2 teaspoons)		0	10g	0	No impact
Mayonnaise - full fat (1 tablespoon)		0.2	14g	0	No impact
Oil - olive (1 tablespoon)		0	15ml	0	No impact
Oil - rapeseed (1 tablespoon)		0	15ml	0	No impact
Bacon - back smoked (2 rashers)		0	70g	0	No impact
Baked Beans (½ tin)		17.9	200g	35.8	Large
Beef Mince (lean, size of a deck of cards - uncooked)		0	100g (uncooked)	0	No impact
Beef steak with bearnaise butter (1 steak)		0.2	150g (cooked)	0.3	No impact
Cannellini beans (2 tablespoons)		15.7	100g	15.7	Medium
Chicken & prosciutto in sauce (½ pack)		1.5	143g	2.2	Small
Chicken mini fillets in gravy (1 pack)		8.1	400g	32.4	Large
Chicken yakitori (4 skewers)		7.8	100g	7.8	Small
Curry - pau bhaji ready meal (½ pack)		9.3	150g	14	Medium

fats   proteins

Carb Awareness Of Everyday Foods

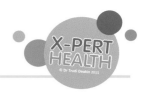

Food/drink	Food image	Carb content per 100g	Portion size	Carbs per portion (g)	Impact on insulin levels
Quorn™ - peppered steaks (1)		5.7	98g	5.5	Small
Veggie burger (1)		17.5	120g	21	Medium
Eggs - scotch (1)		17.5	113g	19.8	Medium
Eggs - chicken (1)		0	80g	0	No impact
Fish - breaded haddock (1 fillet)		28	125g	35	Large
Gammon steak (1)		0	225g	0	No impact
Ham (1 slice)		2	50g	1	No impact
Houmous (1 tablespoon)		15g	60g	9	Small
Lentils - dried red split (uncooked, 1 tablespoon)		56.3	25g (uncooked)	14.1	Medium
Mackerel (1 can)		0	110g	0	No impact
Mackerel (1 smoked fillet)		0	145g	0	No impact
Nuts - almonds (1 small handful)		6.9	25g	1.7	No impact
Nuts - salted peanuts (1 small handful)		10.9	25g	2.7	Small
Pork loin (1 fillet)		0	175g	0	No impact
Prawns (½ pack)		0	83g	0	No impact
Prawns - king (½ pack)		0.8	75g	0.6	No impact
Quiche - tomato & cheese (½ pack)		20.3	165	33.5	Large
Salmon - smoked (1 slice)		0.8g	35g	0.3	No impact

 proteins

www.xperthealth.org.uk

Carb Awareness Of Everyday Foods

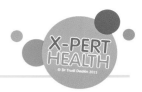

	less than 2g per portion (no impact on insulin levels)		2g to 10g per portion (small impact on insulin levels)		11g to 25g per portion (medium impact on insulin levels)		more than 25g per portion (large impact on insulin levels)

Food/drink	Food image	Carb content per 100g	Portion size	Carbs per portion (g)	Impact on insulin levels
Sardines in tomato sauce (1 can, 95g)		1.5	95g	1.4	No impact
Sausage roll (1 jumbo)		29.5	150g	44.3	Large
Sausages - bacon and cheddar (2)		5.1	84g	4.2	Small
Sausages - chorizo swirl sausage (1)		1.5	100g	1.5	No impact
Sausages - high meat content pork (2)		0.5	133g	0.6	No impact
Tuna (160g can in brine - drained)		0	112g (drained)	0	No impact
Lager - Carling™ 4% (1 can)		2.2	500ml	11.2	Medium
Lager - French premium 4.8% (1 small bottle)		4.4	250ml	11	Medium
Wine - red 13% (1 small glass)		0.8	125ml	1	No impact
Cheese & leek chicken gratin (½ pack)		2.8	170g	4.8	Small
Chicken arrabbiata (1 pack)		12.5	400g	50	Large
Cottage pie (1 pack)		8.2	450g	36.9	Large
Indian meal - jalfrezi and tikka (½ pack)		22	595g	120	Large
Jerk chicken with rice & corn (1 pack)		9.6	380g	36.5	Large
Lasagne - beef (1 pack)		10.7	400g	42.8	Large
Pie - steak & ale (1)		23	200g	46	Large

 proteins   alcoholic drinks   complete meals

Carb Awareness Of Everyday Foods

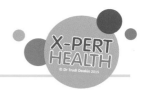

Food/drink	Food image	Carb content per 100g	Portion size	Carbs per portion (g)	Impact on insulin levels
Quorn™ - cottage pie (½ pack)		10	250g	25	Large
Chicken & veg casserole (1 pack)		9.9	440g	43.6	Large
Chicken hotpot (1 pack)		10.5	320g	33.6	Large
Roast pork loin with apple & cider sauce (1 pack)		7.6	390g	29.6	Large
Salmon with potatoes, vegetables & sauce (1 pack)		7.8	385g	30	Large
Sandwich - tuna and sweetcorn (1 pack)		22.3	167g	37.2	Large
Spaghetti carbonara (1 pack)		14.2	400g	56.8	Large
Spinach & ricotta cannelloni (1 pack)		14.9	400g	59.6	Large
Tomato & mozzarella tart (½ tart)		23.4	120g	28.1	Large
Vegetarian spicy three bean enchiladas (½ pack)		21.2	200g	42.4	Large
Fajita seasoning mix (1/8 pack)		41.5	3.75g	1.6	Small
Gravy granules (made up, 125ml)		4.0 (made up)	9g (dry weight)	5.0	Small
Sauce - tikka masala (½ pack)		11.7	185g	21.6	Large

complete meals   miscellaneous

Please note:

1. Changing the portion size may have a different impact on insulin levels. For example: having 2 mixed grain crisp breads may have a medium impact on insulin levels but if you consume 4 this would have a large impact on insulin levels. Having 2 fancy filled chocolates will have a medium impact on insulin levels but having 3 or more will have a large impact.

2. Combining foods that contain carbs may also increase the insulin impact. For example adding 1 teaspoon of jam (9g) to bread (15g) would result in consuming 24g carbs. Adding 1/3 pint of milk (9.6g) to 2 Shredded Wheat™ (27g) will result in consuming 36.6g carbs.

Glycaemic Index

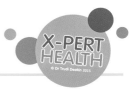

Glycaemic Index is the ranking of carb foods based on their impact on blood glucose levels

The rate that carb foods are released into the blood is compared to glucose. As glucose impacts on blood glucose levels immediately it is given an index of 100. If carb foods release glucose quickly, with an index of above 70, they are called HIGH GLYCAEMIC INDEX foods. Those which break down more slowly, with an index below 55, are called LOW GLYCAEMIC INDEX foods.

Adopting a very low carb dietary approach means that you will be consuming fewer than 50g of carbs per day. Those carbs should come from non-starchy vegetables, low sugar fruit (such as berries and avocado), a small portion of pulses, or dairy food such as whole fat natural yoghurt. All these products are low glycaemic index and so release the glucose more slowly, having a reduced impact on your blood glucose levels.

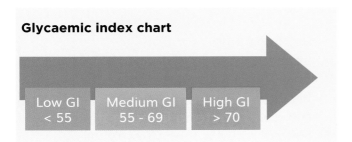

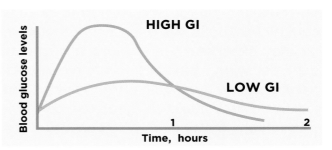

Remember that, although swapping high GI food for lower GI food may help to improve your health, the key is in the AMOUNT of carbs eaten. The table below includes examples of foods that have a high, medium or low GI; but if the carb content is high even the low(er) GI foods will still not be suitable for a very low carb dietary approach.

HIGH GI (quick-releasing) 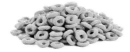	• Glucose / Lucozade™ • Cornflakes™ / Rice Krispies™ • Cheerios™ / Coco Pops™ • Bread (white/wholemeal)	• French bread / Crumpets • Plain biscuits, e.g. Morning Coffee™ • Potatoes (baked/mashed/chips) • Rice (white / brown)
MEDIUM GI 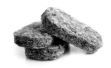	• Sugar / Jam / Fizzy drinks • Ryvita / Basmati rice • Pitta breads / Chapatti • New & Sweet potatoes	• Shredded Wheat™ / Weetabix™ • Rich Tea / Digestive biscuits • Crisps / Popcorn / Muffins • Breads (granary/wholegrain)
LOW GI (slow-releasing) 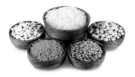	• Muesli* / Porridge* • Milk (cows/soya/almond) • Fromage frais / Yoghurt • Fruit / Vegetables • Pulses (Lentils/Peas/Beans)	• Fruit loaf* / Dried fruit* • Chocolate* / Ice cream* • Pasta (fresh/dried)* • Rye* / Pumpernickel bread* • Seeds / Nuts

* These are examples of foods that have a low GI but still have a high carb content, so are not suitable options for this dietary approach as it will be difficult to include them whilst maintaining a carb intake of less than 50g per day.

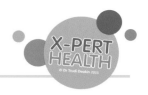

Fibre cannot be digested. It therefore doesn't supply the body with direct energy. A lack of dietary fibre, along with insufficient fluid consumption and sedentary behaviour, can result in constipation. Therefore, to prevent constipation: be as active as possible, keep hydrated and ensure that you consume sufficient fibre. It is currently advised that we should aim for a minimum of 30g fibre every day to decrease the risk of several long-term conditions, but average intake is just 18g each day. If you wish to increase your fibre intake you should aim to do this gradually to build up tolerance. Otherwise you may experience unpleasant side effects such as wind, bloating and diarrhoea. There are two types of fibre; soluble and insoluble. Many fibre-rich foods contain both types of fibre, but one tends to dominate. The two types of fibre have different functions within the body.

Insoluble fibre does not absorb, or dissolve in, water. It passes through our digestive system in close to its original form and is therefore a bulking agent often referred to as "roughage". This can help to increase the speed with which food and waste passes through your gut, helping to prevent and treat constipation.

Soluble fibre escapes digestion and breaks down into short-chain fatty acids in the gut. This provides an excellent source of energy for the cells that line the gut, and for the bacteria that live in the gut too (see page 104). When mixed with water soluble fibre forms a gel-like substance and swells. This "gel" delays digestion, so carb foods that contain soluble fibre tend to be low GI foods. Soluble fibre therefore helps with weight management, as it reduces insulin spikes and helps us to feel fuller for longer.

Adequate consumption of both types of fibre is more likely if people eat real, unprocessed food. The health benefits for each type of fibre are thought to be as follows:

Insoluble fibre - health benefits
- Reduces the calories in food
- May increase the feeling of fullness
- Reduces the risk of haemorrhoids (piles)
- Helps prevent and/or treat constipation

Soluble fibre - health benefits
- Reduces inflammation
- Improves blood glucose, blood insulin and blood fat levels
- Provides nutrition for the gut cells and the good bacteria living in the gut
- Helps create a feeling of fullness
- May help in weight control and reduce the risk of developing several long-term conditions including CVD

A "high fibre" food is classed as having 6g or more of total fibre per 100g. A moderate fibre food has 3g or more. The table overleaf is a quick reference guide of 21 fibrous foods, some of which could support a very low carb dietary approach. At a glance you will see which foods are higher in total fibre, as the table compares 100g of each food. However, how much fibre you actually consume will depend on your portion size. You can also assess which foods are higher in insoluble fibre (e.g. nuts) and soluble fibre (e.g. dark chocolate) using this table. The carb content is shown too so that you can separate low carb foods, (less than 10g carbs/100g) from higher carb foods (e.g. apple, coconut flour, lentils, oats and rice). This doesn't mean that you can't eat or cook with some of these foods, but portions will need to be controlled to keep your carb intake below 50g per day. Oats and rice are best avoided.

Fibre And How It Protects Us

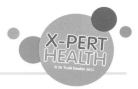

Key:

High fibre: total fibre 6g or more per 100g	Moderate fibre: total fibre 3g to 5.9g per 100g	Low fibre: total fibre less than 3g per 100g
Low carb: total carbs less than 10g per 100g	Moderate carb: 10g to 25g total carbs per 100g	High carbs: total carbs more than 25g per 100g

Food	Food image	Soluble fibre/100g	Insoluble fibre/100g	Total fibre /100g	Total carb /100g
Apple		1	0.5	1.5	12
Artichoke		1	0	1	1.5
Asparagus		1	1	2	2
Avocado		1	4	5	0.5
Berries		0.5	2	2.5	6
Brazil nuts		2.5	5.5	8	3
Broccoli		1.5	2.5	4	2.5
Brussel sprouts		2.5	1.5	4	4
Chia seeds		6	33	39	8
Chocolate (dark 99% cocoa)		16	4	20	8
Coconut flour		2	36	38	21
Flaxseed		15	14	29	1.5
Ground almonds		2	11	13	7
Kidney beans		4.5	4.5	9	13
Lentils		0.5	4.5	5	49
Oats (steel-cut)		4	4	8	64
Rice (wild)		2	4	6	68
Psyllium husk		74	9	83	1.5
Quinoa		3	4	7	49
Spinach		1.5	2.5	4	2
Walnuts		2	4	6	3

All weights based on 100g of raw food product. Different brands may vary

Gut Microbiota

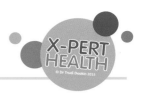

Another important factor that can affect our health is our gut microbiota. A microbe is a living creature that is only visible under a microscope. They exist everywhere: on every surface you touch; on and in every food you eat; in every organ in your body. Just one handful of earth contains more microbes than there are stars in the sky, and one millilitre (1ml) of sea water contains around a million microbes. We have as many microbes in our body as there are human cells – making us as much microbial as we are human!

Thousands of different microbes exist in the gut alone and they are essential to life by:

- Helping us to digest food
- Controlling the amount of energy (calories) we absorb from food
- Maintaining a healthy immune system
- Reducing inflammation (injury) in the body

Bacteria are microbes, and we have a range of bacteria within our gut. Some are beneficial for health and some are not. What separates the good from the bad is how they function:

- **Good bacteria** aid digestion and help to reduce inflammation

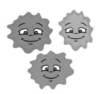

- **Bad bacteria** may do the opposite, increasing inflammation and causing digestive problems such as diarrhoea

Ideally we need a range of beneficial bacteria to reap all the benefits. We call this "diversity" and emerging evidence is helping us understand what we can do to encourage diversity of the good bacteria in our gut.

The composition of our gut microbiota will depend on several factors including:

- Our diet
- The environment we live in
- The medication we take
- Our genetic make-up

Clinical studies have shown that it is possible to increase the number and diversity of beneficial bacteria in our gut, for example we can change our diet to support a healthier gut (see page 105). We may also be able to change some aspects of our environment (see page 106) and the medication (see page 107) we take but we cannot change our genes!

Gut microbiota and body weight

Body weight and body fat seem to be linked with certain types of microbes. Obese individuals have a greater proportion of bad bacteria compared to lean individuals. It appears that some microbes can reduce the absorption of nutrients such as fat and carbs from food. This means that two people could eat the same meal but one would absorb more energy, resulting in a greater chance of weight gain.

A healthy gut microbiota also has the potential to increase:

- your metabolic rate
- levels of hormones that make you feel full
- your body's ability to burn fat for energy

We are starting to learn so much about our gut microbiota and how it can regulate many functions in our body.

Gut Microbiota - Our Diet

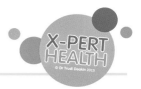

A varied diet leads to lots of different bacteria in our gut, but the types of food we eat will help determine whether we have more good bacteria or more bad bacteria. To promote a healthy microbiota, we need to adopt a diet that leads to a diverse selection of good bacteria.

Prebiotic foods Generally speaking, foods that contain polyphenols (a type of antioxidant) or break down into short-chain fatty acids (SCFAs) feed the good bacteria and encourage diversity of bacteria. Foods that feed the good bacteria are called prebiotic foods. Examples are fruit and vegetables, full fat dairy products, pulses and legumes, polyols, dark chocolate (containing over 80% cocoa solids) and red wine.

Probiotic foods are foods that actually contain live beneficial bacteria and these therefore promote higher levels of good bacteria in the gut. Examples are yoghurt, kefir, sauerkraut, tempeh, kimchi, miso, kombucha, pickles, traditional buttermilk, natto and some types of cheeses such as gouda, mozzarella and cheddar. It is better to consume probiotics from food rather than from supplements because the processing of the supplement may kill the beneficial bacteria. However, if you do decide to take a probiotic supplement and your gut microbiota does improve as a result, you will need to continue to take it long-term. If you discontinue taking the supplement without introducing other pre or probiotics the diversity of your microbes will return to as it was before the supplement was introduced.

Each species of microbe has a preference for specific types of food. This means they are not competing with other microbes for the same things, increasing their chances of survival. To increase these chances further the microbes can send you signals to increase intake of their desired food! We know that a 'junk food diet' increases the number of bad bacteria in the gut, and this could be one reason why many people crave more junk food – the bad bacteria in the gut is telling your brain to eat more of it! The good news is that this negative cycle can be broken ,and once you change your diet and kill off some of the bad bacteria the cravings can disappear!

Foods that promote a healthy microbiota

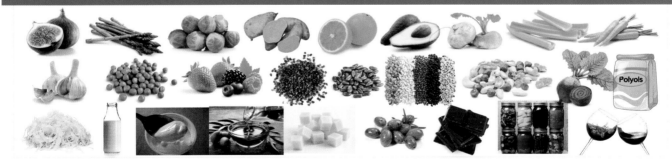

Food that promote an unhealthy microbiota

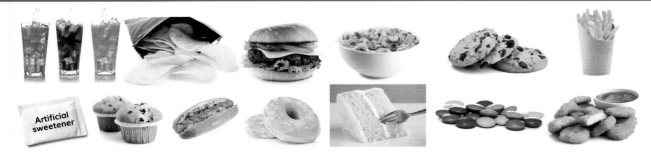

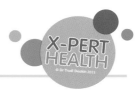

As mentioned previously, there are a number of environmental factors that can have an impact on our gut microbiota. Although these factors are not always the easiest to control or change there are some things we can do to try and help on this front.

How can we change our environment to support a healthy gut microbiota?

Stopping smoking - smoking can increase the 'bad' bacteria in our gut. Stopping smoking may help reverse this and has been shown to increase the diversity of bacteria, potentially helping 'good' bacteria thrive. If you want to give up smoking you can find more information at www.nhs.uk/live-well/quit-smoking/nhs-stop-smoking-services-help-you-quit/

Managing stress - high levels of uncontrolled stress may alter gut microbiota profiles, including lowering the number of potentially beneficial bacteria. Learning to manage stress levels will therefore improve your gut microbiota. See page 56 for more information about stress and how you can reduce it.

Choosing where you live - geography, i.e. where you live or have lived previously, can influence gut bacteria. For example, children born and living in Africa have been found to have more diverse gut bacteria than children in more developed countries. This may be due to dietary differences or exposure to different numbers and types of microbes. Living on a farm can improve the gut microbiota too. It isn't usually possible to change where you live but we can potentially get some similar benefits by getting outside and roaming the countryside where possible, or by having a pet. Not getting too hung up on hygiene and anti-bacterial agents may also help to improve the diversity of good bacteria.

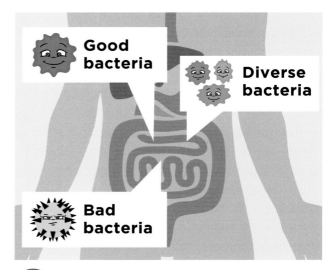

Travel wisely - although travel to overseas destinations may increase exposure to bad or unfamiliar microbes, increasing the likelihood of contracting bacterial or infectious conditions, trying new foods can alter and increase the diversity of our gut bacteria. The tip is to be diligent in where you choose to stay and eat; making sure you choose places where standard hygiene practices are followed.

Reduce exposure to pollution and chemicals - our gut microbiota is exposed to high levels of environmental pollutants on a daily basis, such as food additives and organic pollutants (pesticides and industrial chemicals such as polychlorinated biphenyls "PCBs" and dioxins). Gut bacteria can be sensitive to these environmental pollutants and therefore the diversity and numbers of 'good' bacteria may be affected by exposure. Eating organic and real foods can help to reduce exposure to these chemicals.

Increase levels of physical activity - lack of exercise has been linked to higher levels of potentially 'bad' bacteria in the gut, whereas increased diversity of gut bacteria has been observed in response to exercise. This emphasises the need to ensure sufficient physical activity is undertaken whilst making sure sedentary behaviour is reduced.

Gut Microbiota - Medication

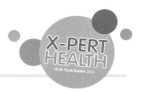

Medication can be essential, but many people also take too much and/or take medication when it is not needed. One of the possible side effects of this can be an impact on our gut microbiota.

How can we change our medication to support a healthy gut microbiota?

• **Antibiotics** can kill off good bacteria in your gut, and it can take two months for the gut to recover from one course of antibiotics. We rely far too much on antibiotics rather than letting the body heal itself. As well as damaging our gut microbiota, overuse may also cause antibiotic resistance. This means if we do have to use them due to a serious bacterial infection, they may become less effective. Do not request antibiotics unless absolutely necessary. If you do have to take antibiotics, you can improve the recovery time of your microbiota with a gut-friendly diet rich in probiotics and prebiotics (see page 105).

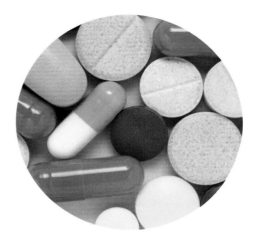

• **Proton pump inhibitors (PPIs), often known as "antacids"**, are medicines taken to reduce the production of acid in the stomach. Therefore they help to control conditions such as acid reflux and heartburn. Altered composition and reduction in diversity of gut microbes have been found in PPI users. It is possible to treat acid reflux and heartburn by making lifestyle changes and losing weight before resorting to medication. A low carb diet has been shown to be successful in some people, enabling omission of antacid medication.

• **Metformin** - this medication is often prescribed to people with polycystic ovary syndrome (PCOS), prediabetes, type 1 and type 2 diabetes. Studies observing the impact of metformin on the gut microbiota are conflicting with some concluding that it promotes a healthy gut whereas others show a decrease in the diversity of bacteria that are present. Clearly more research is needed. The good news is that if you are able to make sufficient lifestyle changes, you may be able to reduce your metformin requirement or omit it altogether.

Did you know that our gut microbiota isn't just affected by things that happen in adulthood?

Factors that affect the microbes in our body start from birth, and include:

• **Caesarean v natural birth** - natural births may increase the diversity of bacteria in an infant's gut. This is thought to be because the baby is exposed to the mother's microbial communities as it passes through the birth canal. However, this does not mean a baby born via caesarean is not exposed to any bacteria before or during birth, as the womb and the mother's skin may also contain many different microbes.

• **Breastfed vs formula-fed** - differences in both composition and diversity of microbes in breastfed and formula-fed infants have been observed. Breastfeeding may help increase bacterial diversity within the infant's gut, as they are exposed to their mother's bacteria in the milk. In turn, this may assist in the development of the infant's immune system. Some formulas however contain probiotics in order to try and promote good bacteria in the infant's gut.

Gut Microbiota - Top Tips

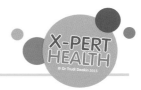

The last few pages have introduced a number of factors that can have an impact on our gut microbiota. Some affect it negatively, resulting in less diversity, less good bacteria and more bad bacteria; and some affect it positively, resulting in more diversity, more good bacteria and less bad bacteria. This information is summarised in the figure below, with the green arrows representing positive factors and the red arrows representing negative factors:

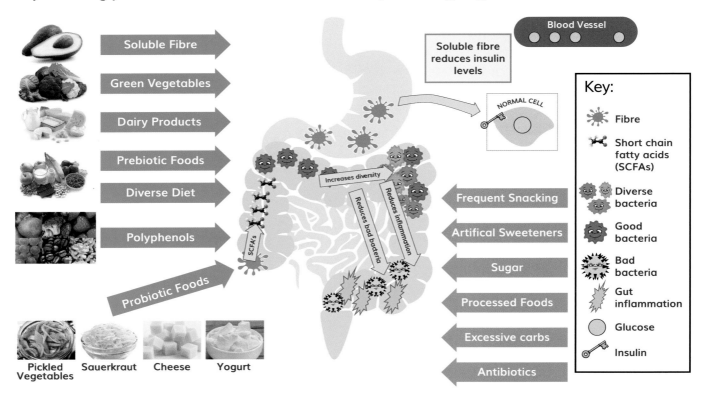

Top tips on how to improve your gut microbiota:

- Eat a diverse diet incorporating foods that support a healthy microbiota; such as vegetables, legumes and beans (though be aware of their carb content when following a very low carb dietary approach), full fat dairy, fermented foods, prebiotics and probiotics

- Minimise intake of artificial sweeteners

- Omit processed junk food and snacks

- Avoid foods with preservatives and additives

- Take action to reduce stress levels

- Make changes to your environment where you can

- Consider getting a pet

- Only take antibiotics and other medications if absolutely necessary. Try making lifestyle changes initially if this is possible

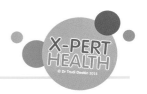

The monitoring health form (on pages 118 and 119) lists the main health results that your healthcare team take into consideration when they monitor your health. If you know and understand your health results and the desired ranges you are more able to make lifestyle changes that improve your health. Ask for your results on a regular basis so that you can see how lifestyle changes have impacted on your health. Remember, these are **your** health results! N.B. Only relevant results will be monitored so don't expect to have all the tests done.

If you have specific questions regarding your own health profile, write them down and discuss these with your healthcare team.

Health indicator

What does it mean?

Weight [kg]

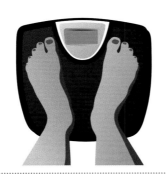

Your body weight is usually measured in kilograms [kg]. If overweight, there are major health benefits from losing even a small amount of weight. Excess weight also makes it harder for your body to use insulin properly (insulin resistance, see pages 8 and 9) and therefore losing weight helps you to control blood glucose levels.

BMI [kg/m²]

BMI Calculator at:
www.nhs.uk/
Tools/PagesHealthy
weightcalculator.aspx

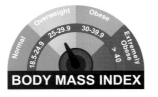

Body Mass Index (BMI) is an assessment of your weight relative to you height. It gives you an indication of whether you are underweight, normal weight, overweight or obese (see page 113).

Waist size [cm] and waist to height ratio (WHtR)

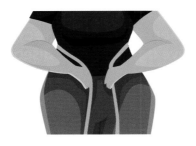

Waist measurements give an indication of whether you are carrying too much weight around your middle. Fat stored centrally increases your risk of developing long-term health problems, such as CVD (see pages 110 and 111). See pages 114 and 115 for more about waist measurements.

Blood Glucose [mmol/l]

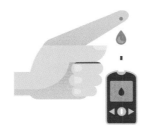

This gives an indication of the amount of glucose in the blood, but only at the time when the blood sample is taken. A reading can be taken when fasting, pre-meal or 1 to 2 hours post meal to monitor blood glucose in the absence or presence of food.

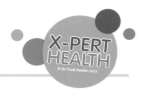

Health indicator		What does it mean?

Glycated haemoglobin "HbA1c" [mmol/mol]

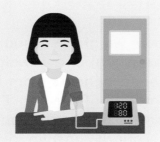

20 mmol/mol

HbA1c 20 mmol/mol — Glucose attached to red blood cells

Good

86 mmol/mol

Bad - too much glucose attached

HbA1c 86 mmol/mol

This blood test measures the amount of glucose that is being carried by the red blood cells in the body. It indicates the average level of glucose in your blood over the last 2 to 3 months. It is the most important tool to help people, especially those with diabetes, understand how well their blood glucose is controlled. A sample is usually taken from a vein in the arm and sent to a lab to be analysed, but devices are now available that enable HbA1c to be determined from a finger prick blood sample.

Blood pressure (BP) [mmHg]

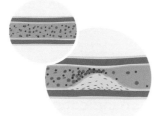

Blood Pressure is the amount of force your blood exerts against the walls of your blood vessels. The first and larger number (systolic BP) is the pressure when the heart pumps the blood into the vessel. The second and smaller number (diastolic BP) is the pressure when the heart is at rest.

Total cholesterol [mmol/l]

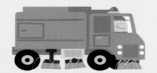

Cholesterol is a waxy substance that is essential to life. It is made in the body but also obtained through diet. It cannot mix with the blood and it is therefore carried by protein transporters (lipoproteins). If the levels of these transporters become unbalanced, or if the transporters become damaged, the risk of CVD increases.

High-density lipoprotein (HDL) [mmol/l]

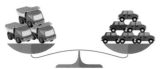

HDL is a cholesterol transporter that mops up excess cholesterol and transports it back to the liver where it is either excreted or recycled. HDL is therefore protective against heart disease. Levels increase with regular physical activity and replacing processed carbs/fats with healthy fats.

Low-density lipoprotein cholesterol (LDL-C) [mmol/l] and particles (LDL-P)

2 people can have the same LDL-C but different LDL-P

LDL-P = 3
LDL-C = 3

LDL-P = 6
LDL-C = 3

LDL-P carry cholesterol to where it is needed. Small dense LDL-P are harmful, causing a build-up of fatty deposits in the lining of blood vessel walls. This increases risk of heart disease and strokes. Large LDL-P are less harmful. Two people can have the same LDL-C, but if one of them has smaller transporters they will need more of them to carry the same load - so they'll have a higher LDL-P. This increases their risk of CVD (see page 73).

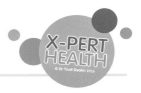

Health indicator **What does it mean?**

Non-HDL cholesterol [mmol/l]

The amount of cholesterol in LDL particles is not measured from a blood test. Instead it is calculated from other blood cholesterol results and this can provide an inaccurate result. There is now a recommendation to monitor non-HDL cholesterol instead of LDL-C.

Non-HDL cholesterol = total cholesterol - HDL cholesterol

Triglycerides (TG) [mmol/l]

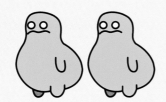

Triglycerides are a type of fat. Raised blood TG levels increase risk of heart disease. Carbs and alcohol can increase levels. Physical activity, eating oily fish, reducing calories from alcohol and carbs and losing weight will help to reduce levels.

Ratios to predict cardiovascular disease (CVD) risk

Total cholesterol (TC) to HDL ratio: This is TC divided by HDL-C. For any given TC level, the more HDL the better. The target is to have a ratio of less than 4.5.

Triglyceride to HDL ratio: Relying on LDL-C alone can be misleading as the cholesterol can either be carried in many small dense particles (harmful) or fewer larger buoyant particles (less harmful). The TG to HDL ratio can give an indication of LDL particle size. Just divide your TG by your HDL-C. A ratio of less than 0.87 is ideal.

This ratio is not reported by UK labs, more information can be found at **www.docsopinion.com/2014/07/17/triglyceride-hdl-ratio/**

Cardiovascular disease (CVD) risk score assessment: QRISK

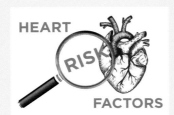

This risk score uses a number of factors such as age, sex, ethnicity, smoking status, diabetes, family history, blood pressure, BMI, total cholesterol to HDL cholesterol ratio, and other health conditions to calculate your risk of having a heart attack or stroke in the next 10 years. If you know the relevant risk factors you can calculate your own risk score at **www.qrisk.org**

Marker of inflammation: C-Reactive Protein (CRP)

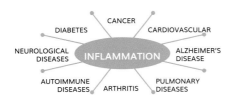

A CRP test is a blood test that measures the general levels of inflammation in your body. Short-term high levels can be caused by infections, but long-term high levels are a risk factor for heart disease, type 2 diabetes and many other conditions.

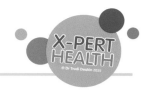

Health indicator   **What does it mean?**

Kidney function tests:

Albumin to creatinine ratio (ACR)

Estimated glomerular filtration rate (eGFR)

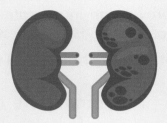

The kidneys filter the blood, removing waste and water to make urine. Tests check how well the kidneys are functioning. The ACR test assesses whether too much protein is leaking into the urine (a sign of kidney damage) and the eGFR test measures how much blood the kidneys are filtering.

Liver function test:

Gamma-glutamyl transpeptidase (GGT)

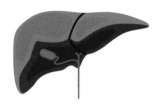

An enzyme found in the liver, GGT is used as a marker for liver disease or excessive alcohol/carb intake. The test provides a very sensitive indicator of the presence of liver diseases, such as fatty liver. Fatty liver can be reversed through lifestyle change, with carb restriction in particular shown to be an effective means of improving this.

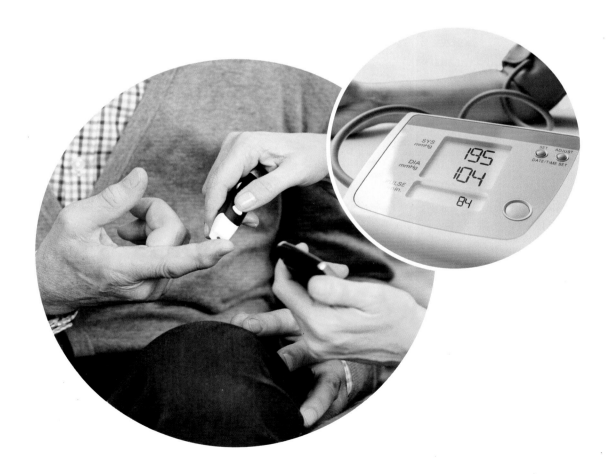

Body Mass Index

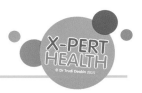

Are you a healthy weight?

Use the chart below to check if you are a healthy weight relative to your height. Find your height and draw a horizontal line across and then find your weight and draw a vertical line. Where the two lines meet will show you what weight section you are in. The World Health Organisation has published different BMI thresholds for Asian people as evidence suggests that people from Asian and other minority ethnic groups are at a higher risk of type 2 diabetes and other health conditions at a lower body mass index (BMI).

Weight St & Lb	7st 12lb	8st 4lb	8st 9lb	9st 1lb	9st 6lb	9st 12lb	10st 3lb	10st 9lb	11st 0lb	11st 6lb	11st 11lb	12st 3lb	12st 8lb	13st 0lb	13st 5lb	13st 11lb	14st 2lb	14st 8lb	14st 13lb	15st 5lb	15st 10lb	16st 2lb	16st 7lb	16st 13lb	17st 5lb	17st 10lb	18st 2lb	18st 7lb	18st 12lb	19st 4lb	19st 9lb
kg	50	52.5	55	57.5	60	62.5	65	67.5	70	72.5	75	77.5	80	82.5	85	87.5	90	92.5	95	97.5	100	102.5	105	107.5	110	112.5	115	117.5	120	122.5	125

Height Ft & In	cm																															
5'0"	152	22	23	24	25	26	27	28	29	30	31	32	34	35	36	37	38	39	40	41	42	43	44	45	47	48	49	50	51	52	53	54
5'1"	155	21	22	23	24	25	26	27	28	29	30	31	32	33	34	35	36	37	39	40	41	42	43	44	45	46	47	48	49	50	51	52
5'2"	157	20	21	22	23	24	25	26	27	28	29	30	31	32	33	34	35	37	38	39	40	41	42	43	44	45	46	47	48	49	50	51
5'3"	160	20	21	21	22	23	24	25	26	27	28	29	30	31	32	33	34	35	36	37	38	39	40	41	42	43	44	45	46	47	48	49
5'4"	163	19	20	21	22	23	24	24	25	26	27	28	29	30	31	32	33	34	35	36	37	38	39	40	40	41	42	43	44	45	46	47
5'5"	165	18	19	20	21	22	23	24	25	26	27	28	28	29	30	31	32	33	34	35	36	37	38	39	39	40	41	42	43	44	45	46
5'6"	168	18	19	19	20	21	22	23	24	25	26	27	27	28	29	30	31	32	33	34	35	35	36	37	38	39	40	41	42	43	43	44
5'7"	170	17	18	19	20	21	22	22	23	24	25	26	27	28	29	29	30	31	32	33	34	35	35	36	37	38	39	40	41	42	42	43
5'8"	173	17	18	18	19	20	21	22	23	23	24	25	26	27	28	28	29	30	31	32	33	34	35	36	36	37	38	38	40	41	41	42
5'9"	175	16	17	18	19	20	20	21	22	23	24	24	25	26	27	28	29	29	30	31	32	33	33	34	35	36	37	38	38	39	40	41
5'10"	178	16	17	17	18	19	20	21	21	22	23	24	24	25	26	27	28	28	29	30	31	32	32	33	34	35	36	36	37	38	39	39
5'11"	180	15	16	17	18	19	19	20	21	22	22	23	24	25	25	26	27	28	29	29	30	31	32	32	33	34	35	35	36	37	38	39
6'0"	183	15	16	16	17	18	19	19	20	21	21	22	23	24	25	25	26	27	28	28	29	30	31	31	32	33	34	34	35	36	37	37
6'1"	185	15	15	16	17	18	18	19	20	20	21	22	23	23	24	25	26	26	27	28	28	29	30	31	31	32	33	34	34	35	36	37
6'2"	188	14	15	16	16	17	18	18	19	20	21	21	22	23	23	24	25	25	26	27	28	28	29	30	30	31	32	32	33	33	34	35
6'3"	191	14	14	15	16	16	17	18	19	19	20	21	21	22	23	23	24	25	25	26	27	27	28	29	29	30	31	32	32	33	34	34
6'4"	193	13	14	15	15	16	17	17	18	19	19	20	21	21	22	23	23	24	25	26	26	27	28	28	29	30	30	31	32	32	33	34

Key: ☐ Underweight ■ Healthy weight ☐ Overweight ☐ Obese ■ Extremely obese

The good news is that losing even a small amount of weight and keeping it off can help to improve your health!

	White/black people	South Asian people
	Body Mass Index (BMI) - kg/m²	
Underweight	less than 18.5	less than 18.5
Healthy weight	18.5 to 24.9	18.5 to 22.9
Overweight	25 to 29.9	23 to 24.9
Obese	30 to 39.9	25 to 34.9
Extremely obese	more than 40	more than 35

Waist Measurements

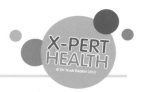

Waist measurements are considered to be a more accurate measure of future health risk than body weight.

Knowing your waist size is more useful than simply knowing if you are a healthy weight, overweight or obese based on your BMI.

This is because the location of your body fat makes a difference to your risk of type 2 diabetes and heart disease. People with excess fat around their waist ("apple" shape) have a greater risk of developing these conditions than people who carry weight on their hips and thighs ("pear" shape).

People who have excess abdominal fat and are in the overweight category for BMI have a greater health risk than people in the obese category who are not carrying excess abdominal fat.

Apple shape vs pear shape

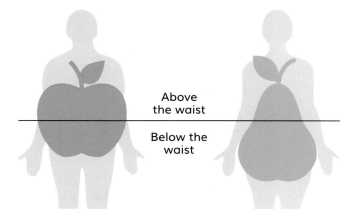

Above the waist

Below the waist

Apple shape

- More fat in and around organs
- Higher risk of weight-related health problems

Pear shape

- Less fat in and around organs
- Lower risk of weight-related health problems

How to measure your waist and assess your health risk

1. Take the measurement without clothes to provide a more accurate measurement

2. Place a tape around the middle point of your waist by doing the following:

   a. find the top of your hip bone (you could mark it with a pen)

   b. find the very bottom of your rib-cage (you could mark it with a pen)

   c. the half-way point between the two marks is the correct position of your waist

   d. place the tape around this point to measure your waist size

   e. try to be relaxed and breathe out gently when reading the measurement. Do not 'suck in' the stomach

   f. write down this number in centimetres (cm) to the nearest 0.1cm

3. Ensure the tape is snug but does not push tightly into the skin

4. Take the measurement twice to check the reading

	SUPER!	ATTENTION!	HIGH RISK!	

Waist Measurements

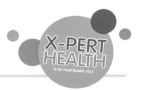

Top tips: If you have difficulty feeling your rib-cage or hip bone (or both), you may find it easier to place your hand, palm down, on your stomach. Place your middle finger on your tummy button and measure your waist just above your index finger.

If you have a prolapse, which has resulted in your tummy button falling below your waist, you may find it easier to slightly bend to the side and measure your waist at the indent.

Consistency is the key! It is therefore advisable to measure your own waist circumference and use the same technique on each occasion.

What does my waist measurement mean?
Use the guidance below to assess your risk

	Healthy waist	**Increased risk**	**High risk**
For Men*	Less than 94cm (about 37 inches)	More than or equal to 94cm (about 37 inches)	More than or equal to 102cm (about 40 inches)
For Women	Less than 80cm (about 32 inches)	More than or equal to 80cm (about 32 inches)	More than or equal to 88cm (about 35 inches)

*For South Asian men a healthy waist measurement is considered to be 90cm (35 inches) or less

Waist to height ratio (WHtR) is an alternative to using waist measurements on their own. It may even be better, as it takes into account that taller people tend to have a larger waist size than smaller people; and the same cut-points apply to everyone.

If your waist size is too large relative to your height, you have an increased risk of future health problems.

How to assess waist to height ratio

1. Measure your waist in cm following the instructions on the previous page
2. Measure your height in cm
3. Divide your waist measurement by your height

Guidelines

- ◼ Ideal = less than 0.50
- ◼ Moderate risk = 0.51 to 0.60
- ◼ High risk = more than 0.60

Your waist should be less than half your height

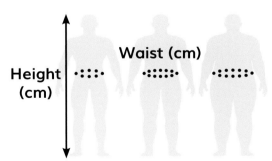

A simple way to test your WHtR is using the string test. Simply cut a piece of string so it is the same height as you (you may need someone to help you with this!), then fold the string in half. If the folded string stretches all the way round your waist, i.e. if the ends overlap at all, then this means your waist is less than half your height!

Tracking Weight

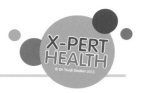

Try to keep a record of your weight and waist circumference, if this is an outcome you are interested in, as this can give a good indicator of your progress. Where possible try to weigh yourself on the same day/time each week, and when measuring waist circumference make sure you use a consistent method.

My height is .... cm

Date	Weight (kg)	Waist size (cm)	Waist to height ratio*	Body fat percentage (%)**

Tracking Weight

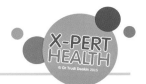

Date	Weight (kg)	Waist size (cm)	Waist to height ratio*	Body fat percentage (%)**

* See page 115 for more details, including how to calculate waist to height ratio

** Some scales estimate this, but it is not essential to record body fat percentage

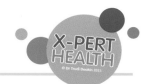

Discuss your individual targets with your healthcare team

Health indicator	Reference range	Date:
Fasting blood glucose (mmol/l)	■ Below 5.6 (normal) ■ 5.5 to 6.9 (prediabetes) ■ 7.0 or above (diabetes)	
HbA1c (mmol/mol) (Average blood glucose)	■ 20 to 41 (normal) ■ 42 to 47 (prediabetes) ■ 48 and above (diabetes)	
Blood pressure (mmHg)	■ Below 120/80 ■ Below 140/90 ■ Above 140/90	
HDL cholesterol (mmol/l)	■ Men: 1.0 or above ■ Women: 1.3 or above	
Triglycerides (mmol/l)	■ Less than 1.7 ■ Between 1.7 - 2.3 ■ More than 2.3	
Triglyceride to HDL ratio	■ Less than 0.87 ■ Between 0.87 - 2.62 ■ More than 2.62	
CVD 10-year risk score assessment QRISK (%)	■ Less than 10 ■ Between 10 - 20 ■ More than 20	
Inflammation: CRP (mg/l)	■ Less than 2.5 ■ Between 2.5 - 5.0 ■ More than 5.0	
Kidney function: 　ACR (mg/mmol) 　eGFR (ml/min/1.73m^2)	■ Men: less than 2.5 & Women: less than 3.5 ■ 60 or more　■ 30 to 59　■ Less than 30	
Liver function: GGT (IU/l)	■ Men: 11 - 50 ■ Women: 7 - 32	

Traffic light coding

■ Target for good health
■ Do I need to take action to improve my health?　　■ What could I do to improve my health?

Monitoring Health

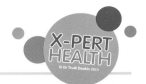

Date:	Date:	Date:	Date:	Date:	Date:

Track your health results over time and see if your lifestyle changes make a difference. You may not be able to obtain all of these health results as some may not be applicable for you.

Tracking Symptoms

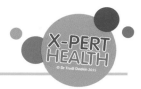

Many people report health improvements above and beyond the things measured in the tests their healthcare team might carry out. It can be useful to record changes in any other factors you might notice, physical or psychological (positive or negative), to help you consider how a very low carb dietary approach might be affecting you. Simple record these in the table below.

Date	Symptom/effect	Comments

We would love to hear about your experiences and value your feedback. If you have anything you would like to share, positive or negative, you can join our free online forum (see the next page for details) or email us at admin@xperthealth.org.uk.